Table of Contents

Beneath the Vein: The Silent Struggles of Blood Disorders

Chapter 1

The Lifeblood of the Human Body

Blood—the very essence of life, coursing through every vein, artery, and capillary in our bodies—does far more than just circulate. It is the highway of life, carrying essential nutrients, oxygen, hormones, and waste products to and from every single cell in the body. Without it, survival would be impossible. This vital fluid is constantly working behind the scenes, invisible yet irreplaceable. Understanding its role and the mechanisms that keep it functioning is essential for grasping how disruptions, like blood disorders, can affect the entire body.

The circulatory system, often referred to as the cardiovascular system, is the complex network of organs and vessels that work in tandem to ensure that blood flows smoothly to where it's needed. It consists of the heart, blood vessels, and the blood itself. The heart serves as the pump, continuously circulating blood through the body, while the blood vessels—arteries, veins, and capillaries—act as conduits that transport this life-sustaining substance to and from every part of our anatomy. But blood is more than just a fluid moving through pipes; it's a dynamic entity with incredible precision, carrying a complex mixture of components designed to perform numerous functions critical for health.

The Composition of Blood: A Delicate Balance

Blood is a complex substance made up of several components, each with its own role to play. The majority of blood, around 55%, is plasma, a yellowish liquid that consists mainly of water but also contains important proteins, electrolytes, hormones, and waste products. Plasma is the medium in which the cellular elements of blood travel. These cells—red blood cells (RBCs), white blood cells (WBCs), and platelets—make up the remaining 45% of blood.

Red blood cells are the most abundant type of blood cell, accounting for nearly 40-45% of the blood's composition. These cells are primarily responsible for carrying oxygen from the lungs to the rest of the body and returning carbon dioxide from the tissues to the lungs for exhalation. Their unique, biconcave shape increases their surface area and flexibility, allowing them to navigate the narrowest capillaries to deliver oxygen effectively.

White blood cells, though fewer in number, play a crucial role in defending the body against infections and diseases. They are part of the immune system, identifying and eliminating harmful invaders like bacteria, viruses, and foreign particles. There are several types of white blood cells, each with specific functions, from producing antibodies to directly attacking pathogens.

Platelets, or thrombocytes, are cell fragments that are key players in blood clotting. When a blood vessel is injured, platelets aggregate at the site to form a plug, helping to seal the wound and prevent excessive bleeding. They work in concert with various proteins in plasma to form a clot, stopping the bleeding and beginning the healing process.

Each of these components must maintain a delicate balance to ensure the circulatory system functions properly. If there is too much or too little of any one component, it can lead to serious health issues. For example, too many red blood cells can cause the blood to become thick and sluggish, while too few can result in insufficient oxygen transport to tissues, leading to anemia.

The Heart: The Unstoppable Pump

At the center of the circulatory system is the heart, a powerful muscle roughly the size of a fist that beats over 100,000 times per day. This tireless pump is responsible for circulating blood throughout the body, maintaining blood pressure, and ensuring that oxygen and nutrients are delivered to organs and tissues. The heart is divided into four chambers: two atria, which receive blood from the body and lungs, and two ventricles, which pump blood out to the lungs and the rest of the body.

The right side of the heart pumps oxygen-poor blood to the lungs, where it is replenished with oxygen, while the left side pumps oxygen-rich blood to the rest of the body. The efficiency of this system is astonishing—at any given moment, the heart is constantly adapting its rhythm and output to meet the demands of the body, whether you are at rest or exerting yourself physically.

Blood Vessels: The Pathways of Life

The network of blood vessels—arteries, veins, and capillaries—forms an intricate system that facilitates the transport of blood throughout the body. Arteries, which carry oxygen-rich blood away from the heart, are thick-walled and elastic, allowing them to withstand the pressure created by the heart's pumping action. The aorta, the largest artery, delivers blood to all parts of the body.

Veins, on the other hand, return deoxygenated blood to the heart. Unlike arteries, veins have thinner walls and rely on one-way valves to prevent blood from flowing backward due to gravity. Capillaries, the smallest blood vessels, form an intricate web that connects the arteries to the veins. These tiny vessels are where the exchange of gases, nutrients, and waste products takes place between the blood and the body's tissues.

The circulatory system is not just about transport; it's a responsive network, adjusting its flow based on the body's needs. For instance, during physical activity, blood flow is redirected to muscles, while during rest, it is concentrated in other areas. Blood vessels dilate or constrict to regulate the distribution of blood, and this level of coordination allows for the dynamic adaptability of the body.

The Vital Functions of Blood

Beyond its role as a transport system, blood is involved in numerous other vital functions:

1. **Oxygen and Nutrient Delivery**: The primary function of red blood cells is to carry oxygen to tissues and organs. Without this delivery system, cells would not be able to produce the energy necessary for survival. Blood also carries essential nutrients, including glucose, amino acids, and fatty acids, to all parts of the body.
2. **Waste Removal**: Blood helps in the removal of metabolic waste products, such as carbon dioxide, urea, and other byproducts. These waste products are transported to organs like the kidneys, lungs, and liver, where they are processed and excreted.
3. **Temperature Regulation**: Blood helps regulate body temperature by absorbing heat from internal organs and transporting it to the skin, where it can be dissipated into the environment. Conversely, blood vessels can constrict to conserve heat in cold conditions.

4. **Immune Response**: White blood cells are the body's primary defense against infection. They recognize and eliminate pathogens, and are an essential part of the immune system's broader response to diseases.
5. **Clotting and Healing**: Platelets and plasma proteins work together to prevent blood loss when a blood vessel is injured. This clotting mechanism ensures that the body can heal from wounds and cuts while minimizing the risk of infection and excessive blood loss.
6. **Hormonal Transport**: Blood also serves as a carrier for hormones, chemical messengers that regulate various bodily functions, from growth and metabolism to reproduction and stress response.

A Delicate Balance: The Precarious Nature of Blood

Despite its incredible efficiency, blood is a delicate system. Any disturbance in the composition or flow of blood can have far-reaching consequences for the body. Blood disorders, which can affect the number of cells or the quality of blood components, pose significant health risks. Conditions like anemia, hemophilia, and blood clots disrupt the delicate balance necessary for optimal body function, leading to symptoms that can range from fatigue and pain to life-threatening complications.

As we embark on this journey to understand blood disorders, it is crucial to appreciate the complexity and precision of the circulatory system. Each component of blood, each vessel, and each beat of the heart plays a vital role in maintaining the body's health. When something goes wrong, it's not just the blood that suffers—it's the entire system. By understanding the lifeblood of the human body, we can better appreciate the significance of these disorders and the profound impact they have on the lives of those affected.

In the chapters ahead, we will explore the common and rare blood disorders that challenge this vital system. From the silent struggles of anemia to the dangerous consequences of blood clots, the journey into the world of blood disorders reveals the fragility of life itself. But it also offers hope through advances in medicine, research, and the resilience of those who live with these conditions every day.

Chapter 2

Red, White, and Everything In Between

The human body is an intricate system, where every part plays a specific role in maintaining balance and harmony. Among the most remarkable and vital components of the body's functions are the blood and its diverse cellular elements. Blood is not just a red liquid circulating within veins and arteries—it is a complex substance composed of many different types of cells and proteins, each contributing to the overall health and functionality of the body. To truly appreciate the critical role of blood, we must explore its many components: red blood cells, white blood cells, platelets, and plasma. These elements work together in perfect harmony, allowing the body to fight disease, transport oxygen, regulate temperature, and heal from injuries. Each component, though unique, is deeply interconnected within the bloodstream's complex journey.

Red Blood Cells: The Carriers of Oxygen

Red blood cells (RBCs), also known as erythrocytes, are by far the most numerous types of blood cell, making up approximately 40-45% of the blood's composition. Their primary function is to transport oxygen from the lungs to the body's tissues and return carbon dioxide, a waste product, from the tissues to the lungs for exhalation. Without these cells, our tissues and organs would quickly become oxygen-starved, resulting in cell death and organ failure.

The structure of red blood cells is crucial to their function. RBCs are biconcave, meaning they have a concave shape on both sides, which increases their surface area and allows them to carry a greater volume of oxygen. This shape also gives them flexibility, enabling them to squeeze through the smallest blood vessels, called capillaries, to deliver oxygen where it is needed. Additionally, red blood cells are devoid of a nucleus, making more room for hemoglobin—the protein responsible for carrying oxygen.

Hemoglobin is a remarkable molecule that binds to oxygen in the lungs and releases it in tissues where oxygen levels are low. Each red blood cell can carry millions of molecules of hemoglobin, which allows for the efficient transportation of oxygen. However, red blood cells do not just deliver oxygen; they also pick up carbon dioxide, a waste product from cellular metabolism, and carry it back to the lungs for exhalation.

The life cycle of a red blood cell is relatively short, lasting about 120 days. During this time, RBCs constantly renew their hemoglobin and undergo wear and tear as they traverse the bloodstream. As they age, they become more rigid and less efficient. The spleen plays a critical role in filtering out old red blood cells, breaking them down and recycling their components, such as iron, to be reused in the production of new RBCs.

White Blood Cells: The Body's Defenders

While red blood cells are essential for oxygen transport, white blood cells (WBCs) serve as the body's primary defense against infection and disease. These cells are far fewer in number than red blood cells, but their impact on the body's immune response is unparalleled. White blood cells, or leukocytes, are responsible for identifying and eliminating pathogens, such as bacteria, viruses, and fungi, as well as protecting the body from harmful substances and abnormal cells, like cancerous cells.

There are several different types of white blood cells, each specializing in specific tasks within the immune system. The primary categories of white blood cells include:

- **Neutrophils**: These are the most abundant type of white blood cell and are the first responders to bacterial infections. They quickly move to the site of infection, where they engulf and digest bacteria through a process known as phagocytosis.
- **Lymphocytes**: These cells include T cells, B cells, and natural killer cells. T cells help coordinate the immune response and can destroy infected cells, while B cells produce antibodies that recognize and neutralize foreign invaders. Natural killer cells are involved in detecting and eliminating abnormal cells, such as cancer cells.
- **Monocytes**: These cells are larger than most white blood cells and are responsible for cleaning up cellular debris and pathogens that neutrophils cannot handle. Once they migrate into tissues, they mature into macrophages, which play an essential role in the immune system's cleanup crew.
- **Eosinophils**: These cells are primarily involved in combating parasitic infections and are also critical in allergic reactions, where they release substances that help control inflammation.
- **Basophils**: Though the least common type of white blood cell, basophils are important for inflammatory reactions, particularly in allergic responses.

They release histamine, which dilates blood vessels and contributes to the symptoms of inflammation.

The immune system's efficiency depends on the proper functioning and coordination of all these white blood cell types. Their ability to differentiate between "self" and "non-self" cells allows the body to fight infections while avoiding harm to its own tissues. White blood cells are constantly circulating in the bloodstream, ready to deploy at the first sign of infection, and they also reside in lymph nodes, spleen, and other parts of the lymphatic system, where they work to identify and eliminate threats.

In addition to protecting the body from harmful invaders, white blood cells also help to regulate inflammation, a process that can become problematic if it is prolonged or excessive. Chronic inflammation is associated with various diseases, including autoimmune disorders, heart disease, and even cancer. Thus, the regulation of white blood cells is crucial for maintaining overall health and preventing disease.

Platelets: The Body's Emergency Response Team

Platelets, or thrombocytes, are the smallest cells in the blood, yet their function is crucial for maintaining vascular integrity and preventing excessive bleeding. Platelets are not full cells but rather cell fragments derived from larger precursor cells called megakaryocytes, which are found in the bone marrow. Despite their small size, platelets are extremely important in the blood clotting process, or hemostasis.

When a blood vessel is injured, platelets are among the first responders to the site of damage. They adhere to the broken edges of the blood vessel, where they release a variety of chemicals that help recruit more platelets to the site of injury. These platelets stick together to form a temporary plug, which is the first step in stopping blood loss. As more platelets accumulate, they interact with clotting factors in the plasma to form a more stable clot, which helps seal the wound and prevents further bleeding.

Platelets are also involved in wound healing. After the clot is formed, the platelets release growth factors that encourage tissue regeneration and repair. This process ensures that the injury site is healed and that normal blood flow is restored. However, while platelets are vital for preventing blood loss, an overactive platelet response can lead to the formation of dangerous blood clots that can block blood vessels, leading to conditions like deep vein thrombosis (DVT) or pulmonary embolism.

Plasma: The Fluid of Life

Plasma, the straw-colored liquid that makes up about 55% of blood, is often seen as the "matrix" in which the cellular components of blood are suspended. However, plasma is far from being just a passive medium—it plays a crucial role in maintaining blood pressure, transporting nutrients, and facilitating the clotting process.

Composed mostly of water (about 90%), plasma also contains a wide array of proteins, hormones, waste products, and electrolytes. Some of the key proteins found in plasma include:

- **Albumin**: The most abundant protein in plasma, albumin helps maintain osmotic pressure and fluid balance within blood vessels. It also serves as a carrier for various substances, such as hormones, vitamins, and drugs.
- **Globulins**: These proteins are involved in immune responses. Immunoglobulins, or antibodies, are a type of globulin that recognizes and neutralizes foreign pathogens, while other globulins transport iron and other nutrients.
- **Fibrinogen**: This protein is essential for blood clotting. When an injury occurs, fibrinogen is converted into fibrin, which forms a mesh-like structure that helps to stabilize the clot and prevent further blood loss.
- **Electrolytes**: Plasma also contains important ions, such as sodium, potassium, calcium, and chloride, which help regulate the body's fluid balance, maintain electrical activity in muscles and nerves, and support various metabolic processes.

Plasma also serves as the medium for transporting a variety of substances throughout the body. It carries nutrients from the digestive system to the tissues, waste products to the kidneys for excretion, and hormones from glands to their target organs. Plasma is also involved in maintaining the body's pH balance and body temperature, ensuring that all systems function efficiently.

The Interplay Between Blood Components

The four major components of blood—red blood cells, white blood cells, platelets, and plasma—are not independent entities but work in a synchronized manner to keep the body functioning smoothly. The precise balance between these components is crucial for maintaining health. An imbalance, such as too few red blood cells (anemia) or too many white blood cells (leukemia), can lead to severe health complications. Likewise, insufficient platelets can result in difficulty clotting, while an overactive clotting response can lead to the formation of harmful blood clots.

Blood is truly a remarkable fluid, with each component playing a unique and vital role in the body's overall health. Whether transporting oxygen to tissues, defending against infection, promoting clotting and healing, or maintaining homeostasis, the components of blood work tirelessly to support life. This complex, yet beautiful, orchestration is what keeps the body in balance and allows it to thrive.

Chapter 3

The Birth of Blood Cells

The human body is a marvel of biological systems, and among the most fascinating is the process by which blood cells are produced. This process, known as **hematopoiesis**, is the foundation for life itself. Blood cells are the lifeblood of our circulatory system, performing countless tasks that keep the body functioning properly. From delivering oxygen to tissues to fighting infections, blood cells are essential to every part of our daily existence. But what happens behind the scenes to ensure that these vital cells are produced in sufficient numbers, and what goes wrong when this process is disrupted?

In this chapter, we will delve into the intricate and fascinating process of hematopoiesis—the creation of blood cells—and explore how this complex system works to maintain a balance of red blood cells, white blood cells, and platelets. We will also look at the disorders that arise when hematopoiesis fails or malfunctions, leading to conditions that can be as simple as anemia or as complex and life-threatening as leukemia.

The Origins of Blood Cells: Bone Marrow as the Factory

Hematopoiesis primarily takes place in the **bone marrow**, a spongy tissue found in the center of certain bones, such as the hips, ribs, and sternum. Bone marrow is often described as the body's "blood cell factory," where the raw materials for blood are continuously being produced. This dynamic process occurs throughout a person's life, ensuring that the blood maintains the right number of cells to carry out its functions.

At the heart of hematopoiesis is a small but incredibly important group of cells known as **hematopoietic stem cells (HSCs)**. These cells are the progenitors of all the different types of blood cells—red blood cells, white blood cells, and platelets. Hematopoietic stem cells are unique in that they have the ability to both **self-renew**, maintaining their population, and **differentiate**, producing various specialized blood cells that will go on to perform specific functions.

Hematopoietic stem cells are multipotent, meaning they can give rise to several types of cells, but they are not unlimited in their differentiation potential. They begin by dividing into **progenitor cells**, which are more specialized and less capable of self-renewal than their parent stem cells. These progenitor cells then further differentiate into **precursor cells**, which eventually mature into the fully functional blood cells we see circulating in the bloodstream.

Stages of Hematopoiesis

The journey of blood cell production begins with **hematopoietic stem cells** in the bone marrow. Through a series of steps, these stem cells become more specialized, ultimately forming the three main types of blood cells: red blood cells, white blood cells, and platelets.

Red Blood Cells: Erythropoiesis

Red blood cells, or **erythrocytes**, are the most numerous cells in the blood and are essential for transporting oxygen. The production of red blood cells, a process known as **erythropoiesis**, begins with a hematopoietic stem cell differentiating into a progenitor cell called an **erythroid progenitor**. These erythroid progenitors begin to mature through several stages. As the precursor cells move through this maturation process, they accumulate hemoglobin, the iron-rich protein that binds oxygen.

The final step of erythropoiesis results in the formation of mature red blood cells. Interestingly, red blood cells are unique in that they lose their nucleus as they mature. This absence of a nucleus maximizes the cell's capacity to carry oxygen by creating more space for hemoglobin.

The production of red blood cells is tightly regulated by **erythropoietin**, a hormone primarily produced by the kidneys. Erythropoietin signals the bone marrow to increase red blood cell production when oxygen levels in the blood are low, ensuring that the body can always meet its oxygen demands.

White Blood Cells: Leukopoiesis

White blood cells, or **leukocytes**, are the key players in the body's immune response. They identify and eliminate pathogens such as bacteria, viruses, and other harmful microorganisms. The process of producing white blood cells is known as **leukopoiesis** and occurs in several stages, depending on the type of white blood cell being produced.

There are several different types of white blood cells, each with its specific function:

- **Granulocytes**: These include neutrophils, eosinophils, and basophils. Granulocytes are involved in the body's response to infection and inflammation. They arise from a common precursor known as the **myeloid progenitor cell**.
- **Agranulocytes**: These include lymphocytes (T cells, B cells, and natural killer cells) and monocytes. Lymphocytes are key players in the adaptive immune response, while monocytes mature into macrophages, which help clear debris and fight infections.

Each type of white blood cell originates from its own precursor cell, but all are ultimately derived from the hematopoietic stem cells in the bone marrow. Lymphocytes are particularly interesting because, after their initial development in the bone marrow, they migrate to other lymphatic tissues, such as the spleen and lymph nodes, to continue their maturation.

The production of white blood cells is regulated by a variety of growth factors, including **colony-stimulating factors (CSFs)** and **interleukins**, which help to stimulate the growth, differentiation, and maturation of the various white blood cell lineages.

Platelets: Thrombopoiesis

Platelets, or **thrombocytes**, are the blood cells responsible for clotting and wound healing. Unlike red and white blood cells, platelets are not true cells but rather fragments of larger precursor cells called **megakaryocytes**, which reside in the bone marrow. The process of platelet production is known as **thrombopoiesis**.

During thrombopoiesis, a megakaryocyte undergoes repeated cycles of DNA replication without cell division, leading to an increase in its size and the eventual fragmentation of its cytoplasm into thousands of smaller pieces. These fragments, now platelets, are released into the bloodstream, where they play an essential role in clotting and wound repair. The process is regulated by **thrombopoietin**, a hormone primarily produced by the liver and kidneys that stimulates the production of megakaryocytes and, consequently, platelets.

Platelets are crucial for preventing excessive bleeding when blood vessels are injured. They gather at the site of injury, adhere to the damaged blood vessel wall, and aggregate to form a clot. They also release substances that aid in the healing process, such as growth factors that stimulate tissue repair.

The Bone Marrow: A Dynamic System

The bone marrow is not a passive structure but a dynamic organ that constantly responds to the body's needs. It is capable of increasing or decreasing the production of blood cells depending on the body's demands. For example, if the body faces an infection, the bone marrow will ramp up the production of white blood cells. If a person loses a significant amount of blood, the bone marrow will quickly produce more red blood cells to restore oxygen levels.

In addition to its role in blood cell production, the bone marrow is also home to other important cells, such as **stromal cells**, which provide structural support to the hematopoietic cells, and **endothelial cells**, which line the blood vessels within the marrow. The marrow is a highly vascularized environment, ensuring that newly produced blood cells are quickly transported into the bloodstream.

When Hematopoiesis Goes Wrong

While hematopoiesis is a finely tuned and essential process, it is not immune to dysfunction. When blood cell production goes awry, it can lead to a variety of blood disorders. These disorders may involve an overproduction of certain cells, such as in leukemia, or an underproduction, as seen in conditions like anemia or thrombocytopenia.

Anemia

Anemia is a condition in which the body does not produce enough red blood cells, leading to insufficient oxygen delivery to tissues. There are many types of anemia, but the most common are **iron-deficiency anemia**, **B12 deficiency anemia**, and **aplastic anemia**, which occurs when the bone marrow fails to produce enough red blood cells.

Leukemia

Leukemia is a cancer of the blood cells, particularly affecting the white blood cells. In leukemia, the bone marrow produces an abnormally high number of immature white blood cells, which crowd out healthy cells and disrupt normal blood function. Leukemia can be acute or chronic, depending on how quickly the abnormal cells proliferate.

Thrombocytopenia

Thrombocytopenia is a condition in which there is a low platelet count, leading to an increased risk of bleeding. This can be caused by a variety of factors, including bone marrow disorders, autoimmune diseases, or certain medications that affect platelet production.

Polycythemia

Polycythemia is a condition in which there is an overproduction of red blood cells, which leads to thicker blood and increased risk of clotting. This can cause problems such as high blood pressure and organ damage due to impaired blood flow.

Conclusion

Hematopoiesis is an extraordinary process that ensures the body's blood cells are continually produced, regulated, and maintained to meet its needs. From the generation of red blood cells that carry oxygen to the production of platelets that stop bleeding, the bone marrow works tirelessly to keep the body in balance. When this process goes awry, however, it can lead to a host of blood disorders that can range from relatively mild to life-threatening. Understanding hematopoiesis not only helps us appreciate the complexity of the human body but also highlights the critical importance of maintaining the health of our blood cell production system.

Chapter 4

The Blood-Brain Barrier

The human body is a complex network of interconnected systems, each working in concert to maintain balance and health. The circulatory system, responsible for transporting blood throughout the body, plays a critical role in this intricate web of interactions. Blood does more than just nourish organs and tissues; it interacts with other systems in ways that are essential for proper function, protection, and communication between different parts of the body. One of the most remarkable, yet lesser-known, systems that blood interacts with is the **blood-brain barrier** (BBB), a highly specialized structure that regulates the flow of substances between the bloodstream and the brain. Understanding the blood-brain barrier is crucial for appreciating how the circulatory system supports not only physical health but also mental and neurological well-being.

In this chapter, we will explore the blood-brain barrier, its vital role in maintaining brain health, and how it interacts with the circulatory system to protect the brain from harmful substances while allowing essential nutrients to pass through. We will also examine how damage to the blood-brain barrier can lead to neurological disorders, and the challenges researchers face in trying to overcome the barrier for medical treatments.

What is the Blood-Brain Barrier?

The blood-brain barrier is a selective, semipermeable membrane that separates the circulating blood from the brain and central nervous system (CNS). It is made up of specialized endothelial cells that line the blood vessels in the brain, as well as glial cells and pericytes, which provide additional structural support and regulate the barrier's permeability. Unlike the blood vessels found in other parts of the body, those in the brain are uniquely designed to restrict the passage of certain substances, while still allowing essential molecules like oxygen, glucose, and amino acids to reach the brain.

The blood-brain barrier is crucial for protecting the brain from harmful toxins, pathogens, and other potentially damaging substances that might circulate in the bloodstream. It also helps to regulate the delicate chemical environment within the brain, ensuring that neurotransmitters, ions, and other molecules are maintained at appropriate levels to support normal brain function. Without this protective barrier, the brain would be vulnerable to infections, inflammation, and toxic compounds, which could result in severe neurological damage.

How the Blood-Brain Barrier Works

The blood-brain barrier's function is primarily based on the tight junctions that exist between the endothelial cells lining the blood vessels. These junctions are different from those found in the rest of the body. In most blood vessels, the endothelial cells are loosely connected, allowing small molecules to pass through and enter surrounding tissues. However, in the brain, these cells are tightly packed together, preventing many substances from slipping through. This selective permeability allows only certain molecules to pass into the brain while keeping out larger, potentially harmful molecules.

The barrier is also aided by **astrocytes**, a type of glial cell that surrounds the blood vessels and helps regulate the exchange of materials between the blood and the brain. Astrocytes release signaling molecules that communicate with endothelial cells, influencing the barrier's permeability and helping maintain its integrity. Additionally, **pericytes**, another type of cell found within the blood-brain barrier, contribute to regulating blood flow within the brain's blood vessels and can influence the barrier's function.

Certain molecules, such as glucose and amino acids, are vital for brain function and must be transported across the blood-brain barrier. These molecules are carried through the endothelial cells by specific transporters that allow their passage into the brain. Oxygen also passes freely through the barrier via simple diffusion, ensuring that brain cells receive the oxygen they need to function. On the other hand, larger molecules, such as proteins and most drugs, are typically unable to cross the barrier without assistance, as they are too large to pass through the endothelial cell junctions.

The Importance of the Blood-Brain Barrier in Health

The blood-brain barrier is essential for protecting the brain from external threats. The brain is one of the most sensitive organs in the body, and any disruption in its delicate balance can lead to serious health consequences. The blood-brain barrier helps maintain this balance by serving as a gatekeeper, allowing the necessary nutrients to enter while keeping out harmful substances, such as:

- **Toxins**: Many harmful substances, such as those produced by infections or environmental pollutants, can be toxic to the brain. The blood-brain barrier prevents these toxins from crossing into the brain and causing damage.
- **Pathogens**: Bacteria, viruses, and fungi that may enter the bloodstream are largely kept out of the brain by the blood-brain barrier. If pathogens manage to breach the barrier, it can lead to conditions such as meningitis or encephalitis, both of which involve inflammation of the brain and can cause serious neurological damage.
- **Immune Cells**: While the immune system is essential for fighting off infections and protecting the body, immune cells, if allowed into the brain, can contribute to inflammation and neurodegeneration. The blood-brain barrier restricts the movement of immune cells, helping to prevent autoimmune responses in the brain.

In addition to protecting the brain from harmful substances, the blood-brain barrier helps regulate the chemical environment of the brain. Neurons in the brain rely on a precise balance of ions, neurotransmitters, and other molecules to communicate with each other and carry out their functions. The blood-brain barrier helps to maintain this balance by tightly controlling the flow of substances into the brain and ensuring that the brain's internal environment remains stable.

Disruptions to the Blood-Brain Barrier

Although the blood-brain barrier is an essential protective mechanism, it is not invulnerable. There are several factors that can lead to damage or dysfunction of the blood-brain barrier, which can, in turn, have serious implications for neurological health.

Injury and Inflammation

Traumatic brain injury (TBI) is one of the most common causes of damage to the blood-brain barrier. A blow to the head or a severe impact can cause the endothelial cells to separate, allowing harmful substances to enter the brain. This can lead to inflammation, oxidative stress, and the accumulation of toxic substances within the brain, all of which can contribute to long-term neurological damage.

In addition to physical injury, inflammation in the brain, as seen in conditions like multiple sclerosis (MS), can also lead to the breakdown of the blood-brain barrier. In MS, immune cells attack the myelin sheath that surrounds nerve fibers, leading to the disruption of the blood-brain barrier and the infiltration of immune cells into the brain. This results in further inflammation and damage to brain tissue.

Chronic Diseases and Aging

Chronic diseases such as hypertension, diabetes, and Alzheimer's disease are also associated with damage to the blood-brain barrier. Over time, high blood pressure and other cardiovascular conditions can weaken the endothelial cells, making the barrier more permeable and allowing potentially harmful substances to cross into the brain. In Alzheimer's disease, the blood-brain barrier becomes compromised, contributing to the accumulation of amyloid plaques in the brain, which are characteristic of the disease and contribute to its progression.

As individuals age, the blood-brain barrier can also become less effective. This age-related decline in barrier function is thought to contribute to the increased vulnerability of older adults to neurological disorders, including cognitive decline and neurodegenerative diseases.

Neurological Disorders and the Blood-Brain Barrier

In diseases like Parkinson's disease, stroke, and epilepsy, the blood-brain barrier may become compromised due to changes in the brain's vascular system. For example, in the case of stroke, the disruption of blood flow to the brain can cause damage to the endothelial cells and lead to leakage of substances that can worsen brain injury. In epilepsy, the blood-brain barrier may become more permeable during seizures, allowing substances to enter the brain that may exacerbate neuronal firing and the risk of further seizures.

Overcoming the Blood-Brain Barrier for Treatment

One of the significant challenges in treating neurological disorders is the presence of the blood-brain barrier. Many medications that could potentially benefit patients with brain disorders cannot effectively cross the blood-brain barrier due to its restrictive nature. This has led to significant efforts to develop ways to deliver drugs and other therapies to the brain.

Several strategies have been explored to overcome this challenge:

- **Nanoparticle-based drug delivery**: Tiny particles that can be engineered to pass through the blood-brain barrier and deliver drugs directly to the brain are an area of active research. These nanoparticles can be designed to carry therapeutic agents, such as chemotherapy drugs or gene-editing tools, and release them at targeted areas in the brain.
- **Focused ultrasound**: This technique uses sound waves to temporarily open the blood-brain barrier, allowing drugs to pass through more easily. While still in the experimental stage, focused ultrasound holds promise for delivering therapies to the brain without causing long-term damage to the barrier.
- **Intranasal delivery**: Certain drugs can be delivered through the nasal passages, which have direct access to the brain through the olfactory nerve. This method bypasses the blood-brain barrier altogether and is being explored as a way to treat conditions like Alzheimer's and Parkinson's disease.
- **Genetic therapy**: Gene therapy, which involves delivering genetic material to cells to treat disease, is also being investigated as a way to bypass the blood-brain barrier. By using vectors, such as viral particles, researchers hope to deliver genes directly to the brain to correct underlying genetic disorders.

Conclusion

The blood-brain barrier is one of the body's most impressive and essential defenses, protecting the brain from harmful substances while ensuring that it receives the nutrients it needs for optimal function. However, this barrier's selectivity can also pose challenges when it comes to treating neurological disorders. Understanding how the blood-brain barrier functions, and how it can be manipulated, is crucial for developing new treatments for brain diseases and improving the quality of life for patients with neurological conditions. The delicate balance the blood-brain barrier maintains is a testament to the sophistication of the body's defenses, highlighting the importance of the circulatory system in supporting overall wellness.

Chapter 5

What is Anemia?

Anemia is one of the most common blood disorders worldwide, affecting millions of people regardless of age, gender, or geographical location. It occurs when the body does not have enough healthy red blood cells to carry adequate oxygen to the tissues. This condition can have a profound impact on an individual's overall health, leading to fatigue, weakness, and a range of other symptoms. While anemia is often seen as a single medical issue, it is, in fact, a broad term that encompasses a variety of conditions, each with its distinct causes, types, and implications.

In this chapter, we will explore what anemia is, its various forms, and the underlying causes that lead to its development. From iron-deficiency anemia to B12 deficiency anemia and beyond, we will break down the types of anemia, how they affect the body, and the treatments available to help manage and resolve this condition. Understanding anemia is not only important for recognizing the symptoms but also for addressing its root causes, as it can be a sign of more serious underlying health issues.

What is Anemia?

At its core, **anemia** is a condition in which the number of red blood cells (RBCs) or the hemoglobin concentration in the blood is lower than normal. Hemoglobin is a protein found in red blood cells that binds to oxygen, allowing the blood to carry it from the lungs to the rest of the body. When there aren't enough red blood cells or when the hemoglobin is insufficient, the body's tissues and organs do not receive the oxygen they need to function properly. This oxygen deprivation can lead to a variety of symptoms, ranging from mild fatigue to more severe complications, depending on the severity of the anemia.

The severity of anemia is classified into mild, moderate, and severe categories, based on the concentration of hemoglobin in the blood. The condition can occur suddenly (acute anemia), as a result of blood loss or another triggering event, or it can develop gradually over time (chronic anemia), often due to nutritional deficiencies, genetic disorders, or chronic diseases.

The symptoms of anemia vary depending on the type and severity but often include:

- **Fatigue**: The most common symptom, caused by insufficient oxygen delivery to muscles and organs.
- **Weakness**: Often accompanied by an overall feeling of tiredness and low energy.
- **Paleness**: A noticeable paleness in the skin, especially in the face or nail beds, is common in people with anemia.
- **Shortness of breath**: Difficulty breathing, especially during physical activity.
- **Dizziness or lightheadedness**: Can occur due to decreased oxygen levels in the brain.
- **Cold hands and feet**: Insufficient blood flow can cause extremities to feel cold.

While these symptoms are common to many types of anemia, the underlying causes and the treatment options differ significantly.

Types of Anemia

Anemia is not a one-size-fits-all condition. It can arise from various underlying factors, each of which can cause distinct forms of the disorder. The most common types of anemia include **iron-deficiency anemia**, **vitamin B12 deficiency anemia**, **folate deficiency anemia**, **sickle cell anemia**, **thalassemia**, and **aplastic anemia**. Below, we will explore the most prevalent types of anemia and their unique causes.

Iron-Deficiency Anemia

Iron-deficiency anemia is the most common type of anemia worldwide. It occurs when the body lacks enough iron to produce sufficient hemoglobin. Iron is a critical component of hemoglobin, the protein that enables red blood cells to carry oxygen. Without enough iron, the body cannot produce enough healthy red blood cells, leading to fatigue, weakness, and other symptoms.

Causes of Iron-Deficiency Anemia:

- **Inadequate dietary intake of iron**: A diet low in iron-rich foods such as meat, legumes, and leafy greens can lead to insufficient iron in the body.

- **Blood loss**: Heavy menstrual periods, gastrointestinal bleeding (such as from ulcers or hemorrhoids), or internal bleeding can lead to significant iron loss.
- **Increased iron needs**: Pregnant women and growing children have increased iron requirements, which, if unmet, can lead to anemia.
- **Malabsorption**: Conditions like celiac disease or inflammatory bowel disease (IBD) can impair the absorption of iron in the digestive tract.

Symptoms of Iron-Deficiency Anemia:

- Fatigue
- Pale skin
- Shortness of breath
- Brittle nails or hair
- Cold hands and feet
- Cravings for non-nutritive substances, such as dirt or ice (known as **pica**)

Treatment for iron-deficiency anemia usually involves increasing dietary iron intake or taking iron supplements. In more severe cases, intravenous iron or blood transfusions may be required.

Vitamin B12 Deficiency Anemia

Vitamin B12 is essential for the production of red blood cells and the proper functioning of the nervous system. **Vitamin B12 deficiency anemia** occurs when the body does not have enough B12 to produce healthy red blood cells, leading to a decrease in the number of red blood cells and impaired oxygen delivery.

Causes of Vitamin B12 Deficiency Anemia:

- **Poor dietary intake**: Vitamin B12 is found primarily in animal products such as meat, eggs, and dairy. Vegetarians and vegans are at higher risk for B12 deficiency.
- **Malabsorption**: Conditions such as **pernicious anemia** (an autoimmune disorder that affects the stomach's ability to absorb B12), **Crohn's disease**, or **celiac disease** can prevent the proper absorption of vitamin B12.
- **Age**: Older adults may have a decreased ability to absorb B12 from food.
- **Certain medications**: Some medications, like proton pump inhibitors or metformin, can interfere with B12 absorption.

Symptoms of Vitamin B12 Deficiency Anemia:

- Fatigue
- Pale or jaundiced skin
- Numbness or tingling in the hands and feet
- Memory problems or cognitive decline
- Difficulty walking or balance issues
- Glossitis (inflamed tongue)

Treatment typically involves B12 injections or high-dose oral supplements. For those who cannot absorb B12 from food, lifelong supplementation may be necessary.

Folate Deficiency Anemia

Folate, also known as vitamin B9, is another essential nutrient for red blood cell production and DNA synthesis. Folate deficiency anemia occurs when the body doesn't have enough folate to produce healthy red blood cells, leading to similar symptoms as vitamin B12 deficiency anemia.

Causes of Folate Deficiency Anemia:

- **Poor dietary intake**: Folate is found in leafy green vegetables, citrus fruits, and fortified foods. A diet lacking these foods can lead to a deficiency.
- **Increased need**: Pregnant women, for instance, require higher levels of folate to support fetal development.
- **Malabsorption**: Conditions that affect the gastrointestinal tract, like Crohn's disease or celiac disease, can impair folate absorption.
- **Excessive alcohol consumption**: Chronic alcohol use can interfere with the body's ability to absorb folate.

Symptoms of Folate Deficiency Anemia:

- Fatigue
- Pale skin
- Shortness of breath
- Irritability
- Diarrhea
- Sore tongue

Folate deficiency anemia is often treated with folic acid supplements and dietary changes. Pregnant women, in particular, are often given folic acid supplements to prevent neural tube defects in the developing fetus.

Sickle Cell Anemia

Sickle cell anemia is a genetic form of anemia that affects the hemoglobin in red blood cells. The condition causes red blood cells to become rigid and shaped like a crescent or sickle, rather than the typical round, flexible shape. These abnormally shaped cells can block blood flow, leading to pain, organ damage, and increased risk of infection.

Causes of Sickle Cell Anemia:

- **Genetics**: Sickle cell anemia is inherited as an autosomal recessive trait. Both parents must carry the sickle cell gene for their child to develop the disease.

Symptoms of Sickle Cell Anemia:

- Episodes of severe pain (called sickle cell crises)
- Fatigue
- Swelling in the hands and feet
- Frequent infections
- Delayed growth in children

Sickle cell anemia cannot be cured, but treatments like pain management, blood transfusions, and medications (such as hydroxyurea) can help manage symptoms and reduce complications.

Aplastic Anemia

Aplastic anemia is a rare but serious form of anemia where the bone marrow fails to produce enough blood cells. This results in a shortage of red blood cells, white blood cells, and platelets. Aplastic anemia can develop suddenly and be life-threatening.

Causes of Aplastic Anemia:

- **Autoimmune conditions**: The body's immune system mistakenly attacks its own bone marrow.
- **Chemical exposure**: Certain chemicals, such as benzene, can damage bone marrow.
- **Radiation or chemotherapy**: These treatments can lead to bone marrow suppression.
- **Viral infections**: In some cases, viral infections, such as hepatitis or Epstein-Barr virus, can lead to bone marrow failure.

Symptoms of Aplastic Anemia:

- Fatigue
- Frequent infections
- Easy bruising or bleeding
- Pale skin

Treatment options include blood transfusions, immunosuppressive therapy, and bone marrow transplants.

Conclusion

Anemia is a multifaceted condition with many causes, ranging from nutritional deficiencies to genetic disorders. Understanding the various types of anemia and their underlying causes is critical to both preventing and managing this condition. While anemia can sometimes be easily treated with dietary changes and supplements, in other cases, it requires more advanced interventions, such as blood transfusions or bone marrow transplants. Regardless of the form it takes, anemia should not be overlooked, as it can be a sign of more serious health problems. Early detection, proper diagnosis, and appropriate treatment can help individuals manage anemia and improve their quality of life.

Chapter 6

Iron-Deficiency Anemia: The Most Common Blood Disorder

Iron-deficiency anemia is by far the most common type of anemia and one of the most widespread nutritional deficiencies worldwide. It is particularly prevalent among women, children, and individuals with certain medical conditions that affect the body's ability to absorb or store iron. Despite its frequency, many people may not immediately recognize the signs of iron-deficiency anemia or understand its long-term implications. In this chapter, we will explore the causes, symptoms, diagnosis, and treatment options for iron-deficiency anemia, offering a comprehensive understanding of this disorder and how it can be managed.

What is Iron-Deficiency Anemia?

Iron-deficiency anemia occurs when the body doesn't have enough iron to produce hemoglobin, the protein in red blood cells responsible for carrying oxygen to tissues and organs. Hemoglobin is composed of iron molecules that bind to oxygen, allowing red blood cells to effectively transport it through the bloodstream. When iron levels are insufficient, the body is unable to produce enough healthy red blood cells, leading to a reduced capacity to deliver oxygen to the body's tissues. As a result, the person may experience fatigue, weakness, and a range of other symptoms associated with insufficient oxygen delivery.

Iron-deficiency anemia is different from other types of anemia in that it specifically relates to a deficiency in iron levels. It can be caused by a variety of factors, including poor diet, blood loss, or conditions that impair the body's ability to absorb iron. It is important to identify and address the root cause of iron deficiency to prevent long-term health complications.

Causes of Iron-Deficiency Anemia

Iron-deficiency anemia is usually the result of one or more factors that lead to a depletion of iron in the body. Below are the most common causes:

1. Inadequate Dietary Intake of Iron

Iron is an essential mineral that must be obtained from the diet. The body cannot produce iron on its own, so it must come from food sources. Iron is found in two forms:

- **Heme iron**, which is found in animal products like red meat, poultry, and fish. This form of iron is more easily absorbed by the body.
- **Non-heme iron**, which is found in plant-based foods like beans, lentils, tofu, spinach, and fortified cereals. Non-heme iron is less efficiently absorbed than heme iron but is still an important dietary source of iron.

A diet lacking sufficient iron-rich foods, particularly for individuals who avoid meat or animal products, can lead to a deficiency over time. Vegetarians and vegans are at a higher risk of iron-deficiency anemia due to their lower intake of heme iron.

2. Blood Loss

Blood loss is one of the most significant causes of iron-deficiency anemia. Any condition or situation that leads to significant blood loss can result in a depletion of iron. Some common causes of blood loss include:

- **Menstrual bleeding**: Women with heavy or prolonged menstrual periods are at increased risk of iron deficiency due to the loss of blood each month.
- **Gastrointestinal bleeding**: Conditions like ulcers, hemorrhoids, gastrointestinal cancer, or inflammatory bowel disease (IBD) can cause internal bleeding that leads to iron loss.
- **Trauma or surgery**: Accidents, injuries, or surgical procedures that involve significant blood loss can also result in a reduction of iron stores.

3. Pregnancy and Growth Spurts

During pregnancy, the body's iron requirements increase significantly to support the growing fetus and placenta. The body's blood volume also expands during pregnancy, which further increases the need for iron. Without adequate iron intake, pregnant women are at high risk of developing iron-deficiency anemia.

Similarly, during periods of rapid growth, such as infancy, childhood, and adolescence, the body requires more iron to support the development of new red blood cells. If these increased needs are not met through diet, iron deficiency can develop.

4. Poor Absorption of Iron

Even if a person consumes enough iron through their diet, certain medical conditions and factors can interfere with the body's ability to absorb iron effectively. Some of the most common conditions that impair iron absorption include:

- **Celiac disease**: This autoimmune disorder damages the small intestine, impairing the absorption of nutrients, including iron.
- **Crohn's disease**: A type of inflammatory bowel disease (IBD) that affects the digestive tract and can lead to malabsorption of nutrients.
- **Gastric surgery**: Surgical procedures that involve the stomach, such as weight-loss surgery or stomach resection, can reduce the surface area available for iron absorption.
- **Chronic use of antacids or proton pump inhibitors**: Medications that reduce stomach acid can interfere with iron absorption since stomach acid is needed to convert iron into a more absorbable form.

5. Increased Iron Requirements

Certain life stages and conditions increase the body's demand for iron. Some of these include:

- **Pregnancy**: As mentioned earlier, pregnant women need more iron to support the developing baby and to compensate for the increase in blood volume.
- **Infancy and childhood**: Rapid growth in young children increases the need for iron.
- **Intense physical activity**: Athletes, especially those involved in endurance sports, may experience a higher turnover of red blood cells and an increased need for iron.

When the body's iron requirements exceed the amount available, iron-deficiency anemia can occur.

Symptoms of Iron-Deficiency Anemia

Iron-deficiency anemia develops gradually, and its symptoms may not be immediately noticeable, particularly in the early stages. However, as the condition worsens, the symptoms become more pronounced. Common symptoms include:

- **Fatigue**: The most common symptom, as the body struggles to deliver enough oxygen to tissues and organs.
- **Weakness**: A general lack of energy, making even simple tasks feel more difficult.
- **Paleness**: A noticeable paleness, especially in the face, hands, or nail beds, due to reduced blood flow and a decrease in red blood cells.
- **Shortness of breath**: Difficulty breathing, especially during physical exertion, as the body lacks sufficient oxygen.
- **Dizziness or lightheadedness**: A feeling of faintness, often experienced when standing up quickly.
- **Cold hands and feet**: Reduced blood flow to extremities can cause a sensation of coldness, particularly in the hands and feet.
- **Brittle nails and hair**: Iron-deficiency anemia can affect the health of your nails and hair, causing them to become dry, brittle, and prone to breakage.
- **Cravings for non-food substances (pica)**: Some individuals with iron-deficiency anemia experience cravings for non-food items, such as dirt, clay, or ice.

If left untreated, iron-deficiency anemia can lead to more severe complications, such as heart problems, impaired immune function, and delayed growth in children.

Diagnosis of Iron-Deficiency Anemia

The diagnosis of iron-deficiency anemia typically involves a combination of a physical examination, medical history, and laboratory tests. A healthcare provider may start by asking about symptoms, diet, and any medical conditions that could contribute to iron deficiency.

The primary diagnostic tool is a **complete blood count (CBC)**, which measures the number of red blood cells and the concentration of hemoglobin. In iron-deficiency anemia, the red blood cells are often smaller and paler than normal, which is a condition known as **microcytic hypochromic anemia**.

Other tests that may be used to diagnose iron-deficiency anemia include:

- **Serum ferritin test**: Ferritin is a protein that stores iron in the body. Low ferritin levels often indicate a deficiency of iron stores.
- **Serum iron and transferrin saturation test**: This measures the amount of circulating iron in the blood and the capacity of transferrin (the protein that transports iron) to bind with iron.
- **Total iron-binding capacity (TIBC)**: This test measures the amount of transferrin in the blood, which can help assess the body's ability to transport iron.
- **Reticulocyte count**: This test measures the number of immature red blood cells in the blood. In iron-deficiency anemia, the number of reticulocytes may be low.

If the cause of iron deficiency is not immediately clear, additional tests may be needed to identify conditions such as gastrointestinal bleeding or malabsorption disorders.

Treatment Options for Iron-Deficiency Anemia

Treatment for iron-deficiency anemia focuses on restoring iron levels and addressing the underlying cause of the deficiency. Common treatment options include:

1. Iron Supplements

The most common and effective treatment for iron-deficiency anemia is oral **iron supplementation**. Iron supplements are available in various forms, including ferrous sulfate, ferrous gluconate, and ferrous fumarate. These supplements help replenish the body's iron stores and improve the production of red blood cells.

It is important to follow the dosage instructions carefully, as taking too much iron can lead to side effects such as constipation, nausea, and abdominal pain. Iron supplements are typically taken with food to reduce gastrointestinal discomfort, although this can slightly reduce absorption. To enhance absorption, iron supplements are often taken on an empty stomach, but this may cause digestive issues for some individuals.

2. Dietary Changes

In addition to supplementation, dietary changes play a crucial role in treating iron-deficiency anemia. Increasing the intake of iron-rich foods can help the body restore its iron stores and prevent further deficiencies. Some good dietary sources of iron include:

- **Heme iron** (more easily absorbed): Red meat, poultry, fish, and shellfish.
- **Non-heme iron**: Beans, lentils, spinach, tofu, quinoa, fortified cereals, and dark leafy greens.

It is also important to include foods rich in **vitamin C**, which enhances the absorption of non-heme iron from plant-based sources. Citrus fruits, tomatoes, bell peppers, and broccoli are all excellent sources of vitamin C.

3. Intravenous Iron

For individuals who cannot tolerate oral iron supplements, or for those with severe iron deficiency that requires rapid intervention, **intravenous (IV) iron** may be administered. This method delivers iron directly into the bloodstream, bypassing the digestive system and allowing for faster replenishment of iron stores.

Treatment of Underlying Causes

If the iron deficiency is due to an underlying health condition, such as gastrointestinal bleeding or malabsorption, treating the root cause is essential to prevent the anemia from recurring. For example:

- **Iron infusion** or **blood transfusions** may be necessary for individuals who experience significant blood loss.
- **Surgical intervention** may be required to treat sources of bleeding, such as ulcers or tumors.

Conclusion

Iron-deficiency anemia is a manageable condition, but it requires early recognition and treatment to avoid long-term health complications. With proper dietary changes, iron supplements, and, when necessary, medical interventions, individuals can regain their iron levels and alleviate the symptoms of anemia. Addressing the underlying causes of iron deficiency is also key to preventing the condition from recurring. By understanding iron-deficiency anemia and the treatment options available, individuals can take proactive steps to improve their health and well-being.

Chapter 7

Vitamin B12 Deficiency: The Silent Culprit

Vitamin B12, also known as cobalamin, is an essential water-soluble vitamin that plays a crucial role in the body's overall health, particularly in the production of red blood cells and the proper functioning of the nervous system. Unlike other vitamins, the body does not naturally produce vitamin B12, which means it must be obtained through dietary sources or supplements. For individuals who are unable to absorb or utilize vitamin B12 effectively, a deficiency can develop, leading to a condition known as **Vitamin B12 deficiency anemia**.

This chapter will explore the causes, symptoms, and diagnostic challenges of B12 deficiency, shedding light on the potential long-term effects of neglecting this critical deficiency and providing a roadmap for diagnosis and treatment. Often referred to as the "silent culprit," B12 deficiency can go unnoticed for a long time because its symptoms develop gradually and can be mistaken for other conditions. It is only with a deeper understanding and careful attention that the true nature of this deficiency can be identified and managed.

What is Vitamin B12 Deficiency?

Vitamin B12 is involved in several important bodily functions, including:

- **Red blood cell production**: B12 helps in the formation of red blood cells in the bone marrow. A deficiency impairs the production of these cells, leading to megaloblastic anemia, a condition in which red blood cells are abnormally large and less effective at carrying oxygen throughout the body.
- **Neurological health**: B12 plays a vital role in maintaining the health of the nervous system, particularly the myelin sheath that covers and protects nerve fibers. Without adequate B12, nerve function is disrupted, leading to neurological symptoms such as tingling or numbness in the hands and feet, memory problems, and mood disturbances.
- **DNA synthesis**: The vitamin is also essential for the proper synthesis of DNA, which is necessary for the production and function of all cells in the body.

When a person's B12 levels drop too low, the consequences can be wide-ranging, affecting the body's blood cells, nervous system, and overall vitality. The gradual onset of symptoms often makes it difficult for individuals and healthcare providers to pinpoint B12 deficiency early on.

Causes of Vitamin B12 Deficiency

There are several reasons why a person might become deficient in vitamin B12. These causes can be broadly categorized into dietary, absorption-related, and medical factors.

Dietary Deficiency

`The most common cause of B12 deficiency is inadequate intake of the vitamin through the diet. Vitamin B12 is primarily found in animal products such as meat, fish, dairy, and eggs. As a result, individuals who follow strict vegetarian or vegan diets are at an increased risk of developing a deficiency if they do not take steps to include fortified foods or supplements.

While plant-based foods do not contain vitamin B12, there are some fortified plant-based alternatives available, including fortified cereals, plant-based milk, and nutritional yeast. However, those who avoid all animal products and do not supplement with vitamin B12 may develop a deficiency over time, especially if they do not consume enough of these fortified foods.

Absorption Issues

For the body to effectively use the vitamin B12 from food, several steps must occur, and any disruption in these processes can lead to a deficiency. The absorption of B12 involves a complex process:

- **Intrinsic factor**: A glycoprotein produced in the stomach is essential for vitamin B12 absorption. Intrinsic factor binds with B12 in the small intestine, allowing it to be absorbed by the body.
- **Stomach acid and enzymes**: The stomach produces acid and enzymes that help release vitamin B12 from food. Without sufficient stomach acid, the vitamin cannot be freed from the protein in food.
- **Small intestine health**: The absorption of B12 takes place in the ileum, the final portion of the small intestine. Any damage to this area can impede B12 absorption.

Several conditions can affect the body's ability to absorb vitamin B12:

- **Pernicious anemia**: This autoimmune disorder is one of the most common causes of B12 deficiency. It occurs when the immune system attacks the cells in the stomach that produce intrinsic factor, rendering the vitamin B12 unable to be absorbed properly.
- **Gastrointestinal disorders**: Conditions like **Crohn's disease, celiac disease**, and **gastrectomy** (surgical removal of part or all of the stomach) can reduce the body's ability to absorb B12 from food. Additionally, individuals with **acid-reducing medications** such as proton pump inhibitors (PPIs) or H2 blockers may experience reduced stomach acid, leading to difficulty releasing B12 from food.
- **Helicobacter pylori infection**: This bacterial infection can affect the stomach lining and interfere with the absorption of vitamin B12.

Age-Related Factors

As people age, their stomachs tend to produce less acid, which can reduce the ability to absorb vitamin B12. The elderly are particularly susceptible to B12 deficiency, and it is not uncommon for older adults to be diagnosed with pernicious anemia. Furthermore, the aging process can lead to a decline in intrinsic factor production, which is necessary for B12 absorption.

Medications and Medical Conditions

Certain medications and medical treatments can also interfere with the body's ability to absorb or utilize vitamin B12. These include:

- **Metformin**: A common medication used to treat type 2 diabetes has been associated with reduced B12 absorption.
- **Long-term use of proton pump inhibitors (PPIs) or H2 blockers**: These medications, which are used to reduce stomach acid, can interfere with the stomach's ability to release vitamin B12 from food.
- **Chloramphenicol**: An antibiotic that can inhibit the production of red blood cells, interfering with B12 utilization.
- **Surgical removal of parts of the stomach or small intestine**: This can result in a reduced surface area for nutrient absorption.

Symptoms of Vitamin B12 Deficiency

Vitamin B12 deficiency often develops gradually, and its symptoms may not be immediately recognized, particularly because they can mimic those of other health issues. The condition can affect various parts of the body, leading to both physical and neurological symptoms.

Hematologic Symptoms

The most immediate effect of B12 deficiency is on the blood. As mentioned earlier, vitamin B12 is crucial for the production of red blood cells. When B12 is lacking, the bone marrow produces large, immature red blood cells known as **megaloblasts**, which cannot function properly. This leads to **megaloblastic anemia**, a condition in which the red blood cells are oversized and incapable of carrying sufficient oxygen. Common hematologic symptoms include:

- **Fatigue**: A sense of constant tiredness or exhaustion, as the body struggles to produce healthy red blood cells to deliver oxygen to tissues.
- **Weakness**: Generalized weakness that can make normal daily tasks more difficult.
- **Paleness**: Reduced red blood cell count can cause an overall pallor, especially noticeable in the skin and gums.
- **Shortness of breath**: Even minor physical exertion may leave the individual feeling winded or out of breath.

Neurological Symptoms

Because vitamin B12 plays such an important role in the nervous system, a deficiency can lead to serious neurological symptoms. These may develop slowly and worsen over time if the deficiency is left untreated:

- **Numbness or tingling**: Often referred to as **paresthesia**, individuals may feel a "pins and needles" sensation, typically in the hands, feet, or legs.
- **Memory problems**: B12 deficiency can affect cognitive function, leading to forgetfulness, difficulty concentrating, and in severe cases, dementia-like symptoms.
- **Mood disturbances**: Depression, irritability, and anxiety have been linked to B12 deficiency. This is partly because vitamin B12 is involved in the synthesis of neurotransmitters that regulate mood.
- **Difficulty walking**: Severe B12 deficiency can damage the nervous system to the point where it affects coordination and balance, leading to unsteadiness or difficulty walking.
- **Glossitis**: A swollen, inflamed tongue, which may become smooth and sore, is a common sign of B12 deficiency.

Other Symptoms

Other symptoms of B12 deficiency can include:

- **Sore mouth or ulcers**: People may experience a painful, inflamed tongue or mouth sores.
- **Heart palpitations**: The body may compensate for reduced red blood cell counts by increasing heart rate.
- **Jaundice**: Yellowing of the skin and eyes, caused by the breakdown of abnormal red blood cells.

Diagnosing Vitamin B12 Deficiency

Because the symptoms of vitamin B12 deficiency can be vague and overlap with many other conditions, diagnosing it can be challenging. A healthcare provider will begin with a thorough medical history and physical examination, considering dietary habits, existing medical conditions, and medications that may be affecting B12 absorption. The primary tests used to diagnose B12 deficiency include:

- **Serum B12 levels**: A blood test that measures the amount of vitamin B12 in the blood. Low levels indicate a deficiency, but it is important to note that certain factors (such as kidney disease or pregnancy) can influence B12 levels, so further testing may be required.
- **Methylmalonic acid (MMA)** and **homocysteine levels**: These markers can be elevated in the presence of B12 deficiency, even if serum B12 levels are borderline. Elevated levels of MMA and homocysteine are indicative of impaired B12 metabolism.
- **Complete blood count (CBC)**: This test may reveal the presence of megaloblastic anemia, with large, immature red blood cells.

In some cases, additional testing, such as **intrinsic factor antibody tests** or **gastric biopsy,** may be required if pernicious anemia or other underlying causes are suspected.

Treatment of Vitamin B12 Deficiency

The treatment of vitamin B12 deficiency primarily involves replenishing the body's B12 stores through supplementation. Depending on the severity of the deficiency and the underlying cause, treatment may include:

Oral Supplements

In cases of mild to moderate deficiency, oral vitamin B12 supplements are typically recommended. These can come in various forms, including tablets, sublingual (under the tongue) tablets, and chewable tablets. The dosage will vary depending on the individual's needs, with higher doses often prescribed for those with malabsorption issues.

Vitamin B12 Injections

For individuals with more severe B12 deficiency or those who are unable to absorb vitamin B12 through the digestive system (such as in pernicious anemia or after gastric surgery), **B12 injections** are often recommended. These injections deliver the vitamin directly into the bloodstream, bypassing the digestive tract.

Dietary Modifications

Individuals with dietary deficiencies, particularly those who follow vegan or vegetarian diets, are advised to incorporate more vitamin B12-rich foods into their meals. These include animal products like meat, poultry, eggs, and dairy, or fortified plant-based foods like nutritional yeast, soy milk, and breakfast cereals.

Addressing Underlying Conditions

If a medical condition such as pernicious anemia or a gastrointestinal disorder is the cause of the B12 deficiency, appropriate treatment for that condition will also be necessary. This might include medications to treat the autoimmune condition or surgery for digestive issues.

Conclusion

Vitamin B12 deficiency is often referred to as the "silent culprit" due to its gradual onset and nonspecific symptoms that can be easily overlooked. However, with proper diagnosis and treatment, B12 deficiency is highly manageable. Early intervention is crucial to prevent irreversible damage to the nervous system and to address the blood-related issues caused by a lack of B12. By increasing awareness of the causes, symptoms, and treatment options for this common yet often overlooked condition, individuals can take proactive steps to ensure their health and well-being.

Chapter 8

Megaloblastic Anemia: The Role of Folate

Megaloblastic anemia is a type of anemia characterized by the production of abnormally large, immature red blood cells, known as megaloblasts, in the bone marrow. This condition is often caused by deficiencies in **vitamin B12** or **folate (vitamin B9)**, two essential nutrients that are crucial for the proper formation of red blood cells and the overall health of the body. While vitamin B12 deficiency is perhaps the more widely known cause, **folate deficiency** plays an equally significant role in the development of megaloblastic anemia. This chapter will explore the critical role that folate plays in the body, the causes and effects of folate deficiency, and the ways in which this deficiency impacts the body's ability to produce healthy red blood cells.

What is Folate and Why is it Important?

Folate, also known as vitamin B9, is a water-soluble B-vitamin that is involved in a wide range of physiological functions, particularly in the **formation of DNA** and the **production of red blood cells**. As a coenzyme, folate is essential for the synthesis and repair of DNA, making it crucial for cell division and the growth of new cells. This is particularly important in rapidly dividing tissues, such as the bone marrow, where blood cells are continuously produced.

Folate also plays an essential role in the metabolism of homocysteine, an amino acid that, when elevated, can increase the risk of cardiovascular disease. By converting homocysteine into methionine, folate helps maintain a healthy balance of amino acids and supports cardiovascular health.

The Mechanisms of Folate in Red Blood Cell Production

The process of red blood cell production, known as **erythropoiesis**, occurs in the bone marrow. During this process, folate is essential for the production of **nucleic acids (DNA and RNA)**, which are necessary for the division and maturation of red blood cells. When folate levels are low, the process of erythropoiesis is disrupted, leading to the formation of large, abnormal red blood cells that are incapable of functioning properly. These **megaloblasts** are typically released from the bone marrow prematurely, leading to a condition known as **megaloblastic anemia**.

In addition to its role in red blood cell production, folate is crucial for **cellular metabolism** and **tissue growth**. Deficiencies in folate not only lead to issues with the production of red blood cells but can also affect the function of other rapidly dividing cells, such as those in the gastrointestinal system and the skin. This is why folate deficiency can lead to a variety of symptoms affecting multiple systems in the body.

Causes of Folate Deficiency

Folate deficiency is often the result of **insufficient intake, impaired absorption**, or **increased requirements**. Let's explore each of these potential causes in more detail.

Inadequate Dietary Intake

The most common cause of folate deficiency is an inadequate intake of folate-rich foods. Folate is naturally found in many foods, including:

- **Leafy green vegetables** (such as spinach, kale, and broccoli)
- **Fruits** (such as oranges, bananas, and avocados)
- **Legumes** (such as lentils, beans, and chickpeas)
- **Whole grains** (such as fortified cereals and brown rice)
- **Nuts and seeds**

A diet low in these foods can lead to a folate deficiency, especially in populations that have limited access to fresh fruits and vegetables. Individuals with poor eating habits, those with restricted diets (e.g., vegetarians or vegans), or those who consume processed foods with few folate-rich ingredients are at risk of inadequate folate intake.

Malabsorption Issues

Even if an individual consumes enough folate in their diet, certain medical conditions can impair the body's ability to absorb and utilize the vitamin. Conditions that can lead to folate malabsorption include:

- **Celiac disease**: A chronic autoimmune disorder that damages the small intestine and impairs nutrient absorption.
- **Crohn's disease**: A type of inflammatory bowel disease (IBD) that can affect the small intestine and reduce folate absorption.

- **Alcoholism**: Chronic alcohol consumption can lead to damage to the gastrointestinal tract, impairing the absorption of folate, as well as other vital nutrients.
- **Gastrectomy or gastrointestinal surgery**: Surgical procedures that remove part of the stomach or small intestine can reduce the area available for nutrient absorption.

In addition, some medications can interfere with the absorption or utilization of folate. For example, drugs used to treat **epilepsy**, such as **phenytoin** and **valproate**, as well as certain **chemotherapy medications**, can impair folate metabolism.

Increased Folate Requirements

Certain life stages and medical conditions can increase the body's need for folate. For example:

- **Pregnancy**: During pregnancy, the body requires more folate to support the growth and development of the fetus. Folate is particularly important during the early stages of pregnancy for the formation of the baby's neural tube, which later develops into the brain and spinal cord. Pregnant women are often advised to take folic acid supplements to ensure they meet these increased needs and to prevent **neural tube defects** in the baby.
- **Infancy and childhood**: Growing children also have higher folate requirements to support rapid cell division and tissue growth.
- **Chronic conditions**: Certain chronic conditions, such as **hemolytic anemia**, **chronic kidney disease**, and **cancer**, can increase the body's need for folate, as they require more red blood cells and cellular repair.

People in these categories may require higher amounts of folate to prevent deficiency, particularly if they have an underlying condition or insufficient dietary intake.

Symptoms of Folate Deficiency

The symptoms of folate deficiency can be subtle at first but tend to worsen over time if left untreated. The most notable symptoms are related to **megaloblastic anemia**, which impacts the body's ability to produce sufficient and healthy red blood cells.

Hematologic Symptoms

- **Fatigue**: The reduced ability of red blood cells to carry oxygen throughout the body leads to feelings of tiredness, weakness, and fatigue.
- **Paleness**: Insufficient healthy red blood cells can lead to a pale complexion, especially in the skin and inside the mouth.
- **Shortness of breath**: As a result of the anemia, individuals may experience breathlessness even with mild physical exertion.
- **Dizziness and lightheadedness**: The lack of sufficient oxygen delivery to the brain can cause dizziness or a sensation of lightheadedness.
- **Heart palpitations**: The heart may work harder to compensate for the lack of red blood cells, leading to rapid heartbeats or palpitations.

Neurological Symptoms

While folate deficiency is primarily linked to hematologic symptoms, it can also affect the nervous system, although to a lesser extent than vitamin B12 deficiency. Symptoms may include:

- **Cognitive disturbances**: Difficulty concentrating, forgetfulness, and trouble thinking clearly can result from a lack of folate.
- **Mood changes**: Folate plays a role in the production of neurotransmitters, so a deficiency can contribute to symptoms of depression, irritability, or anxiety.
- **Neurological issues**: In severe cases, a folate deficiency can result in peripheral neuropathy, causing symptoms such as tingling, numbness, and weakness, particularly in the hands and feet.

Oral Symptoms

People with folate deficiency may also experience **glossitis**, a condition where the tongue becomes swollen, red, and sore. The tongue may appear smooth and glossy, and there may be a loss of papillae (the small bumps on the surface of the tongue). Mouth sores and ulcers can also develop.

Gastrointestinal Symptoms

Folate deficiency can cause gastrointestinal symptoms, including **diarrhea**, **loss of appetite**, and **nausea**, due to the rapid turnover of cells in the gastrointestinal tract.

Diagnosis of Folate Deficiency

Diagnosing folate deficiency typically involves a combination of clinical evaluation, blood tests, and a review of the patient's medical history and dietary habits. The following tests are commonly used:

- **Serum folate test**: A blood test that measures the level of folate in the bloodstream. Low levels indicate a deficiency, but this test does not always reflect tissue folate levels.
- **Red blood cell folate**: This test measures the amount of folate in red blood cells and provides a more accurate reflection of long-term folate status.
- **Complete blood count (CBC)**: A CBC can reveal megaloblastic anemia, with abnormally large red blood cells, which is indicative of a folate deficiency.

Further testing may be necessary to rule out other conditions that may cause similar symptoms, such as **vitamin B12 deficiency** or **iron deficiency anemia**.

Treatment of Folate Deficiency

The primary treatment for folate deficiency is to increase folate intake either through diet or supplements. The specific treatment depends on the severity of the deficiency and any underlying medical conditions.

Folate Supplements

For individuals diagnosed with folate deficiency, folate supplements are typically prescribed. These supplements are available in various forms, including oral tablets, liquid formulations, or injectable forms for those with absorption issues.

Dietary Changes

In addition to supplementation, individuals are encouraged to consume more folate-rich foods. For those with a dietary deficiency, increasing the intake of **leafy greens**, **fortified cereals**, **fruits**, and **legumes** can significantly improve folate levels.

If the folate deficiency is secondary to another medical condition, such as **malabsorption issues**, treatment of the underlying condition will also be necessary. This might include medication for gastrointestinal disorders, alcohol cessation programs, or adjustments to current medications.

Conclusion

Folate deficiency and the resulting megaloblastic anemia can have significant effects on the body's ability to produce healthy red blood cells. By understanding the causes, symptoms, and treatment options for folate deficiency, individuals can take proactive steps to prevent and manage this condition. Early diagnosis and intervention are key to preventing complications and ensuring optimal health, particularly for vulnerable populations such as pregnant women, the elderly, and those with chronic illnesses.

Chapter 9

A Deeper Look at Anemia of Chronic Disease

Anemia is often seen as a condition caused by nutritional deficiencies, such as iron or vitamin B12. However, there is another type of anemia that is commonly linked to underlying chronic diseases, a condition referred to as **Anemia of Chronic Disease (ACD)**, or sometimes **Anemia of Inflammation**. Unlike other forms of anemia that are typically caused by a lack of essential nutrients, ACD occurs as a consequence of chronic illness or inflammation. Chronic conditions like **chronic kidney disease (CKD)**, **cancer**, **rheumatoid arthritis**, and other inflammatory disorders can lead to changes in the body's iron metabolism, red blood cell production, and the regulation of erythropoiesis (the process of creating new red blood cells), resulting in a persistent low red blood cell count.

This chapter will delve into the mechanisms, causes, and symptoms of anemia of chronic disease, as well as the impact of various long-term illnesses on blood health. We will also examine treatment approaches and how healthcare providers manage this common and often overlooked form of anemia.

What is Anemia of Chronic Disease (ACD)?

Anemia of Chronic Disease is a type of anemia that typically occurs in the context of chronic illnesses and long-term inflammatory conditions. It is often characterized by **normocytic** or **microcytic anemia**, which means that the red blood cells may appear normal or slightly smaller than usual in size, but their ability to carry oxygen is compromised. The key feature of ACD is that it is not due to a deficiency in nutrients such as iron, vitamin B12, or folate, but instead results from **alterations in the body's response to inflammation** and chronic disease.

This form of anemia is particularly common in individuals with conditions that cause prolonged inflammation, infection, or tissue damage, including chronic kidney disease, cancer, rheumatoid arthritis, and other autoimmune disorders. Unlike other forms of anemia that can be corrected by supplementing missing nutrients, ACD often requires addressing the underlying disease and its associated inflammatory processes.

The Mechanisms of Anemia of Chronic Disease

The pathophysiology of anemia of chronic disease is complex, involving various immune and inflammatory pathways. While the exact mechanisms are still being studied, several key factors contribute to the development of this condition:

The Role of Inflammation

One of the main factors behind ACD is chronic inflammation, which leads to changes in how the body handles iron and produces red blood cells. When the body is fighting chronic infection or disease, **inflammatory cytokines** like **interleukin-6 (IL-6)** and **tumor necrosis factor-alpha (TNF-alpha)** are released into the bloodstream. These cytokines have several effects on iron metabolism and erythropoiesis:

- **Iron sequestration**: Inflammation triggers the liver to produce a protein called **hepcidin**, which plays a central role in iron metabolism. Hepcidin inhibits the absorption of iron from the digestive tract and limits the release of iron from stores in the liver and spleen. This results in **iron sequestration**—the trapping of iron in storage sites, where it cannot be utilized by the bone marrow to produce red blood cells. Despite the presence of sufficient iron in the body, it becomes unavailable for red blood cell production.
- **Impaired erythropoiesis**: Chronic inflammation disrupts the production of red blood cells in the bone marrow. In particular, the production of **erythropoietin**, a hormone that stimulates the bone marrow to make red blood cells, is often decreased or suppressed during prolonged inflammation. Additionally, inflammation alters the normal functioning of stem cells in the bone marrow, hindering their ability to differentiate into mature red blood cells.

Reduced Erythropoiesis

In individuals with chronic disease, particularly those with kidney disease or cancer, there is often a **dysregulated erythropoietin response**. Erythropoietin (EPO) is a hormone produced by the kidneys that signals the bone marrow to increase red blood cell production in response to low oxygen levels. In chronic kidney disease, the kidneys are unable to produce adequate amounts of erythropoietin due to damage to the renal tissues. This leads to a deficiency in

EPO, which contributes to decreased red blood cell production and the development of anemia.

Moreover, cytokines released during inflammation, such as **interleukins** and **TNF-alpha**, can also suppress the bone marrow's ability to produce red blood cells. This means that even though the body may have enough iron, vitamins, and minerals for red blood cell production, the chronic inflammation itself hinders the ability of the bone marrow to respond to the body's need for more red blood cells.

Shortened Red Blood Cell Lifespan

In people with chronic diseases, the lifespan of red blood cells is often reduced. In a healthy person, red blood cells typically live for around 120 days before they are removed by the spleen. However, in individuals with chronic inflammation, red blood cells tend to break down more rapidly due to the effects of cytokines and immune system activation. This leads to a higher turnover of red blood cells, and in the setting of poor erythropoiesis, it can further contribute to a low red blood cell count.

Chronic Diseases Associated with Anemia of Chronic Disease

Several chronic diseases are strongly associated with anemia of chronic disease. The following are some of the most common conditions that can lead to this form of anemia:

Chronic Kidney Disease (CKD)

Anemia is one of the most common complications of chronic kidney disease. The kidneys are responsible for producing erythropoietin (EPO), the hormone that stimulates red blood cell production. In CKD, the damaged kidneys produce less erythropoietin, leading to a decrease in red blood cell production. Additionally, CKD often results in inflammation, which further suppresses erythropoiesis and causes iron retention, leading to anemia. Therefore, anemia in CKD is primarily due to both insufficient erythropoietin production and inflammatory effects.

Cancer

Cancer and its treatments can also contribute to anemia of chronic disease. Certain cancers, particularly those affecting the bone marrow (such as leukemia or lymphoma), directly impact the production of red blood cells. Additionally, chemotherapy and radiation therapy, while targeting cancer cells, also damage normal cells in the bone marrow, further impairing red blood cell production. Inflammatory cytokines released by cancer cells or in response to tumors can also disrupt iron metabolism and contribute to anemia.

Inflammatory Disorders (e.g., Rheumatoid Arthritis)

Rheumatoid arthritis (RA) and other autoimmune diseases cause chronic inflammation that leads to the development of anemia of chronic disease. In RA, the immune system attacks the joints, leading to inflammation that triggers the release of pro-inflammatory cytokines. These cytokines, such as IL-6 and TNF-alpha, interfere with erythropoiesis and iron metabolism, contributing to the development of anemia.

Chronic Infections

Long-term infections, particularly those that persist over time (such as tuberculosis or HIV), can also lead to ACD. Chronic infections often trigger the immune system to produce inflammatory cytokines that suppress erythropoiesis, decrease iron availability, and contribute to the development of anemia.

Cardiovascular Disease

Chronic cardiovascular conditions, including heart failure and chronic ischemic heart disease, can result in anemia of chronic disease. Similar to kidney disease, heart disease can lead to reduced oxygen delivery to tissues and a compensatory increase in erythropoietin production, but the inflammatory environment in cardiovascular disease can inhibit red blood cell production and lead to iron dysregulation, worsening anemia.

Symptoms of Anemia of Chronic Disease

The symptoms of anemia of chronic disease are generally similar to those of other forms of anemia and may include:

- **Fatigue**: A hallmark symptom of anemia, caused by insufficient oxygen delivery to the body's tissues.
- **Weakness**: Due to the decreased ability of red blood cells to carry oxygen, muscles and other tissues do not receive the oxygen they need, leading to generalized weakness.

- **Paleness**: Anemia can cause a noticeable paleness in the skin, particularly around the face and the mucous membranes, such as the gums.
- **Shortness of breath**: Due to reduced oxygen-carrying capacity, individuals may experience difficulty breathing, even with mild exertion.
- **Dizziness and lightheadedness**: These symptoms occur when the brain is not receiving enough oxygenated blood.

In cases of chronic kidney disease or cancer, patients may also experience additional complications like swelling in the legs or abdomen, and in patients with inflammatory conditions like rheumatoid arthritis, joint pain and stiffness may be more pronounced.

Diagnosis of Anemia of Chronic Disease

Diagnosing anemia of chronic disease typically involves several steps, including blood tests and an assessment of the patient's medical history. Key diagnostic tools include:

- **Complete Blood Count (CBC)**: A CBC test will show a low hemoglobin level, and the red blood cells may appear **normocytic** or **microcytic**. In ACD, the hemoglobin levels tend to be mildly reduced, and the red blood cells may have a normal or smaller-than-usual size.
- **Iron Studies**: Tests measuring **serum iron**, **ferritin**, and **transferrin saturation** will reveal low iron availability but normal or high iron stores in the body. This is because inflammation leads to iron sequestration in the liver and spleen.
- **Erythropoietin levels**: Measurement of erythropoietin can help determine if low EPO levels are contributing to anemia, particularly in chronic kidney disease.

Treatment of Anemia of Chronic Disease

The treatment of anemia of chronic disease depends largely on the underlying condition causing the inflammation. Key approaches may include:

1. **Addressing the underlying disease**: The most effective treatment for ACD is often to treat the chronic disease itself. For example, in rheumatoid arthritis, immunosuppressive drugs may be used to reduce inflammation, while in chronic kidney disease, the use of **erythropoiesis-stimulating**

agents (ESAs) like **epoetin alfa** may help stimulate red blood cell production.
2. **Iron supplementation**: In some cases, iron supplementation may be used, though its effectiveness is limited by the body's inability to utilize iron due to inflammatory processes.
3. **Blood transfusions**: In severe cases, when anemia leads to life-threatening symptoms, blood transfusions may be necessary to stabilize the patient and provide immediate relief.
4. **Management of comorbidities**: For patients with multiple chronic conditions, such as heart failure and kidney disease, comprehensive management is necessary to improve overall health and reduce the burden of anemia.

Conclusion

Anemia of chronic disease is a complex and often misunderstood condition that can arise as a result of long-term illnesses or inflammation. Understanding its mechanisms, associated diseases, and treatment options is crucial for managing this form of anemia and improving the overall health and quality of life for affected individuals. By addressing the underlying causes of inflammation and restoring normal blood cell production, patients can often achieve better outcomes and minimize the impact of anemia on their daily lives.

Chapter 10

Diagnosing Anemia: From Blood Tests to Treatment Plans

Anemia, a condition in which the body lacks enough healthy red blood cells to carry adequate oxygen to tissues, can be caused by a variety of factors. Whether due to iron deficiency, chronic disease, vitamin deficiencies, or genetic disorders, anemia is a multifaceted condition that requires precise diagnosis to determine the underlying cause and provide effective treatment. In this chapter, we will explore the comprehensive process of diagnosing anemia, from the initial assessment of symptoms to the advanced blood tests and diagnostic tools used by healthcare providers. We will also discuss how a correct diagnosis leads to the creation of tailored treatment plans that aim to address both the anemia and its root cause.

Step 1: Recognizing the Symptoms

Anemia often develops gradually, and its symptoms can range from mild to severe. In some cases, it may be so subtle that individuals do not recognize they are unwell. The first step in diagnosing anemia begins with **recognizing symptoms** and evaluating a patient's medical history. Common signs and symptoms of anemia include:

- **Fatigue and weakness**: These are the most common and telltale symptoms of anemia. As red blood cells carry oxygen to tissues and organs, a reduction in their number leads to decreased oxygen supply, leaving the body feeling tired and weak.
- **Paleness of the skin and mucous membranes**: When blood oxygen levels are low, the skin may appear paler than usual, especially in the face, lips, and nail beds.
- **Shortness of breath**: Anemia may lead to difficulty breathing, even with light physical exertion, as the body tries to compensate for the lack of oxygen in the blood.
- **Dizziness or lightheadedness**: Insufficient oxygen in the brain can cause feelings of dizziness, particularly when standing up suddenly.
- **Chest pain and headache**: As the body's tissues, including the heart and brain, become deprived of oxygen, some individuals may experience chest pain or frequent headaches.

- **Cold hands and feet**: Reduced blood flow and oxygenation can result in extremities feeling cold to the touch.

Recognizing these symptoms is crucial for physicians to consider anemia in the differential diagnosis. However, these signs are not exclusive to anemia, and many other conditions, such as chronic heart failure or hypothyroidism, can present similarly.

Step 2: Initial Medical Examination

After a patient presents with symptoms that may suggest anemia, the next step is typically a **medical examination**. This includes taking a detailed medical history and conducting a physical exam to assess the severity of the symptoms and look for signs of anemia. During the exam, the healthcare provider may check:

- **Heart rate and blood pressure**: Anemia often leads to a faster heartbeat (tachycardia) or a drop in blood pressure, especially when standing (orthostatic hypotension).
- **Pale skin**: A visual inspection of the skin and mucous membranes, including the inside of the mouth, can help assess paleness indicative of anemia.
- **Nail and hair condition**: In cases of iron deficiency anemia, nails may become brittle, and hair may thin.
- **Splenomegaly or hepatomegaly**: An enlarged spleen or liver may indicate an underlying cause of anemia such as a blood disorder or chronic disease.

Once a preliminary assessment is made, the physician will order blood tests to confirm the diagnosis and identify the specific type of anemia. Blood tests are the cornerstone of anemia diagnosis, and they help clinicians determine the severity of the anemia and uncover its underlying cause.

Step 3: Blood Tests and Their Role in Diagnosis

Blood tests are essential for diagnosing anemia and differentiating between the various types. The following tests are commonly used in diagnosing anemia:

1. Complete Blood Count (CBC)

The **Complete Blood Count (CBC)** is the first and most important test used to diagnose anemia. It provides a broad overview of the blood's components, helping clinicians assess the number, size, and concentration of red blood cells. Key measurements from the CBC include:

- **Hemoglobin (Hb)**: This is the protein in red blood cells responsible for carrying oxygen. Low hemoglobin levels indicate anemia.
- **Hematocrit (Hct)**: This test measures the proportion of blood made up of red blood cells. A low hematocrit indicates that the body has fewer red blood cells than normal.
- **Red Blood Cell Count (RBC)**: A direct count of the red blood cells. A low RBC count suggests anemia.
- **Mean Corpuscular Volume (MCV)**: MCV measures the average size of red blood cells. It is used to classify anemia as microcytic (small red blood cells), normocytic (normal-sized red blood cells), or macrocytic (large red blood cells), which can help determine the cause.
- **Mean Corpuscular Hemoglobin (MCH)**: This reflects the average amount of hemoglobin in a red blood cell. A low MCH indicates iron-deficiency anemia, whereas a high MCH may suggest a vitamin B12 or folate deficiency.
- **Red Blood Cell Distribution Width (RDW)**: RDW measures the variation in size of red blood cells. A high RDW may indicate a mixed population of red blood cells, which can be seen in conditions like anemia due to vitamin deficiencies or chronic disease.

The CBC is helpful in confirming anemia and providing initial clues about its type.

2. Iron Studies

Iron studies are particularly helpful in diagnosing iron-deficiency anemia. These tests measure various components of the body's iron metabolism, including:

- **Serum Iron**: Measures the amount of iron in the blood. Low levels suggest a deficiency in iron.
- **Ferritin**: Ferritin is a protein that stores iron in the body. Low ferritin levels are a strong indicator of iron deficiency anemia, while normal ferritin levels can suggest anemia due to chronic disease or other causes.
- **Total Iron-Binding Capacity (TIBC)**: TIBC measures how much iron the blood can carry. High TIBC can indicate iron deficiency, while low TIBC may suggest anemia of chronic disease or inflammation.

- **Transferrin Saturation**: This measures the percentage of transferrin (an iron-carrying protein) that is bound with iron. Low transferrin saturation suggests a lack of available iron for red blood cell production.

Iron studies help healthcare providers identify whether the anemia is due to an iron deficiency or another cause.

3. Vitamin B12 and Folate Levels

Vitamin B12 and folate are essential for red blood cell production, and deficiencies in either of these nutrients can lead to **megaloblastic anemia**. Blood tests measuring levels of **serum vitamin B12** and **serum folate** are useful for diagnosing this type of anemia. In cases of **pernicious anemia**, an autoimmune condition that affects vitamin B12 absorption, **antibodies to intrinsic factor** can also be tested.

4. Reticulocyte Count

The **reticulocyte count** measures the number of immature red blood cells in the bloodstream. A high reticulocyte count suggests that the bone marrow is actively producing red blood cells in response to a deficiency or anemia. However, a low count can indicate that the bone marrow is not responding appropriately, which may occur in conditions like anemia of chronic disease or bone marrow disorders.

5. Coombs Test (Direct Antiglobulin Test)

If the physician suspects that anemia may be due to an **autoimmune hemolytic disorder** (such as **hemolytic anemia**), a **Coombs test** may be conducted. This test checks for the presence of antibodies that are attacking and destroying red blood cells prematurely. The **direct Coombs test** is used to detect antibodies attached to red blood cells, while the **indirect Coombs test** checks for antibodies in the bloodstream that could cause red blood cell destruction.

6. Bone Marrow Biopsy

In rare cases, if the cause of anemia is unclear after the blood tests, a **bone marrow biopsy** may be performed. This involves taking a sample of bone marrow from the hipbone to examine the production of red blood cells. Bone marrow biopsies are often used to diagnose serious conditions like leukemia, myelodysplastic syndromes, or other bone marrow disorders.

Step 4: Identifying the Underlying Cause

Once anemia is confirmed through laboratory testing, the next crucial step is to identify the **underlying cause** of the anemia. Anemia can result from a variety of conditions, including:

- **Nutritional deficiencies** (iron, vitamin B12, folate)
- **Chronic diseases** (kidney disease, cancer, rheumatoid arthritis)
- **Blood loss** (from gastrointestinal bleeding, heavy menstruation, surgery, or trauma)
- **Hemolysis** (destruction of red blood cells due to autoimmune conditions or infections)
- **Bone marrow disorders** (such as leukemia or aplastic anemia)
- **Inherited conditions** (such as sickle cell anemia or thalassemia)

Identifying the underlying cause of anemia is vital, as it guides treatment decisions and helps healthcare providers understand how best to address the condition.

Step 5: Developing a Treatment Plan

Once anemia is diagnosed and its underlying cause is determined, the next step is to develop a **treatment plan** tailored to the patient's specific needs. Treatment options may include:

- **Iron supplementation** for iron-deficiency anemia, either in oral or intravenous form.
- **Vitamin B12 or folate supplementation** for deficiencies in these nutrients.
- **Erythropoiesis-stimulating agents (ESAs)** for individuals with chronic kidney disease or cancer-related anemia.
- **Blood transfusions** in severe cases of anemia to immediately increase red blood cell count and oxygen delivery.
- **Immunosuppressive therapy** for autoimmune hemolytic anemia.
- **Bone marrow transplant** or **chemotherapy** for patients with bone marrow diseases or hematologic cancers.

Treatment plans will also address any comorbidities or contributing factors, such as managing chronic diseases or treating gastrointestinal bleeding.

Conclusion

The diagnosis of anemia is a comprehensive process that involves recognizing symptoms, conducting a thorough medical exam, and performing detailed blood tests. Once diagnosed, identifying the underlying cause of anemia is crucial for effective treatment and improving patient outcomes. By understanding the diagnostic process and the array of medical tools available, clinicians can accurately identify the type and cause of anemia, allowing for the development of personalized treatment plans that target both the anemia and its root causes.

Chapter 11

The Blood Clotting Mechanism

Blood clotting is a vital process that protects the body from excessive blood loss following injury, ensuring the repair and healing of damaged tissues. It is a complex mechanism involving a series of coordinated events where blood transforms from a liquid state to a gel-like clot. The clotting process, known as **hemostasis**, prevents excessive bleeding by sealing off broken blood vessels. However, while this process is essential for survival, an imbalance can lead to either excessive clotting, which can result in dangerous thrombosis, or insufficient clotting, leading to uncontrolled bleeding. This chapter will explore the intricate steps of the blood clotting mechanism, the role of platelets and coagulation factors, and how the body maintains a delicate balance to ensure proper clot formation.

The Importance of Blood Clotting

Blood clotting, or coagulation, is necessary whenever there is injury to blood vessels, such as a cut or rupture. Without this mechanism, even small wounds could lead to fatal blood loss. The body's ability to form a clot depends on the interaction between various elements in the blood, including platelets, plasma proteins, and the vessel walls. Hemostasis can be divided into three major phases:

1. **Vascular spasm (Vasoconstriction)**: The immediate response to blood vessel injury is constriction of the vessel walls to reduce blood flow to the affected area.
2. **Platelet plug formation**: Platelets, or thrombocytes, are small, colorless cell fragments that play a key role in clotting. They adhere to the site of injury and to each other, forming a temporary "platelet plug."
3. **Coagulation (Fibrin clot formation)**: The final stage involves a cascade of enzymatic reactions, leading to the conversion of fibrinogen, a soluble plasma protein, into insoluble fibrin strands. These strands weave through the platelet plug, forming a stable clot that prevents further blood loss and facilitates tissue healing.

Platelets: The Primary Players in Clot Formation

Platelets are critical components of the clotting process. These small, disc-shaped cell fragments are produced in the bone marrow by megakaryocytes and circulate in the bloodstream. Though they lack a nucleus, platelets contain various granules with proteins and enzymes essential for the clotting process. When blood vessels are injured, platelets become activated and initiate the clotting process.

Platelet Activation and Adhesion

When blood vessels are damaged, the underlying tissue layers, including collagen and other proteins, are exposed to the circulating blood. Platelets immediately begin to **adhere** to the exposed collagen and other substances at the site of injury. This is facilitated by a protein called **von Willebrand factor (vWF)**, which acts as a bridge between the platelets and the damaged vessel wall.

Once platelets adhere to the injury site, they become **activated** and undergo a series of changes. Platelets release chemical signals stored in their granules, including **ADP (adenosine diphosphate), thromboxane A2**, and **serotonin**, which attract more platelets to the site and promote further platelet aggregation. Additionally, platelets change shape, becoming spiky and sticky, which enhances their ability to stick to each other and form a growing **platelet plug**.

Platelet Aggregation

Platelet aggregation is the process by which activated platelets stick together, forming a "platelet plug" to temporarily seal the damaged vessel. The aggregation process is driven by **fibrinogen**, a plasma protein that binds to **GPIIb/IIIa receptors** on the surface of activated platelets, linking them together. This aggregation is critical for forming the initial "barrier" to prevent excessive blood loss while the clotting cascade occurs to stabilize the clot.

The Coagulation Cascade: A Complex Series of Reactions

While platelets form a temporary plug at the injury site, the **coagulation cascade** is the process by which the body forms a more permanent clot. This cascade involves a series of complex biochemical reactions that result in the conversion of the plasma protein **fibrinogen** into **fibrin**, which solidifies the clot. The coagulation cascade is typically divided into three stages: the **extrinsic pathway**, the **intrinsic pathway**, and the **common pathway**.

The Extrinsic Pathway (Tissue Factor Pathway)

The extrinsic pathway is the first step in the coagulation cascade and is triggered when there is injury to the vascular wall. When the blood vessels are damaged, the tissue underlying the vessel wall is exposed. This tissue contains a protein called **tissue factor (TF)**, also known as **factor III**. Tissue factor combines with **factor VII** from the plasma to form an active enzyme complex, which activates **factor X**, the central protein in the coagulation cascade.

The Intrinsic Pathway (Contact Activation Pathway)

The intrinsic pathway is a series of reactions triggered by the exposure of blood to the negatively charged surface of the damaged vessel or the platelet plug. The key components of the intrinsic pathway are several coagulation factors present in the plasma, including **factor XII, factor XI, factor IX**, and **factor VIII**. This pathway amplifies the signal from the extrinsic pathway and activates **factor X** in the common pathway.

The Common Pathway

The common pathway is where the extrinsic and intrinsic pathways converge. Once activated, **factor X** combines with **factor V** to form the **prothrombinase complex**. This complex catalyzes the conversion of **prothrombin** (factor II) into **thrombin**. Thrombin plays a crucial role in the coagulation process by converting **fibrinogen** into **fibrin**.

Fibrin Formation and Clot Stabilization

Fibrinogen is a soluble protein present in plasma that acts as a precursor to fibrin, the fibrous protein that forms the meshwork of the clot. When thrombin is produced, it cleaves fibrinogen into fibrin monomers, which then aggregate and form long strands. These strands intertwine to create a dense fibrin mesh that stabilizes the platelet plug.

At the same time, thrombin activates **factor XIII**, which cross-links the fibrin strands, further strengthening and stabilizing the clot. This process creates a solid, stable clot that effectively seals the wound and prevents further blood loss. The clot also provides a scaffold for tissue repair and healing to occur underneath the clot.

Anticoagulants: Balancing Clot Formation and Preventing Excessive Clotting

While blood clotting is essential for wound healing and preventing hemorrhage, it must be tightly regulated to prevent excessive clotting, which can lead to thrombosis—a dangerous condition that can block blood flow and cause conditions such as heart attacks, strokes, or deep vein thrombosis. The body has built-in mechanisms to **regulate clotting** and prevent the formation of abnormal or excessive clots.

Several natural anticoagulants exist within the bloodstream to control the clotting process. These include:

- **Antithrombin**: This protein inhibits the action of thrombin and other coagulation factors, such as factor Xa, preventing the coagulation cascade from continuing unchecked.
- **Protein C and Protein S**: These proteins work together to deactivate factors Va and VIIIa, inhibiting clot formation and promoting clot resolution.
- **Tissue factor pathway inhibitor (TFPI)**: This protein inhibits the extrinsic pathway by binding to the tissue factor-factor VII complex, preventing the activation of factor X.

These anticoagulants help maintain a balance in the blood clotting process, ensuring that clots form only when necessary, and they dissolve when the clotting stimulus has passed.

Disorders of Blood Clotting: Hemophilia and Hypercoagulability

Disorders of the blood clotting system can have serious health implications. **Hemophilia**, for example, is a genetic disorder in which certain coagulation factors, such as factor VIII or factor IX, are deficient or absent. As a result, individuals with hemophilia have difficulty forming stable clots, which leads to excessive bleeding after injury or surgery. Hemophilia is often classified into two types—**Hemophilia A**, caused by a deficiency of factor VIII, and **Hemophilia B**, caused by a deficiency of factor IX.

On the other hand, **hypercoagulability** refers to a state in which the blood is more prone to clotting, increasing the risk of conditions such as deep vein thrombosis (DVT), pulmonary embolism, or stroke. Hypercoagulability can be inherited or acquired and often involves abnormalities in clotting factors, the presence of **antiphospholipid antibodies**, or conditions such as **protein C deficiency**.

Conclusion

The blood clotting mechanism is an intricate and finely tuned process that protects the body from excessive blood loss following injury. The involvement of platelets, coagulation factors, and regulatory proteins ensures that clots form quickly and efficiently while preventing excessive or inappropriate clotting. However, disorders in this delicate system can lead to either excessive bleeding, as in hemophilia, or excessive clotting, as in hypercoagulable states. Understanding the blood clotting mechanism is crucial for diagnosing and treating clotting and bleeding disorders, helping to maintain a balance that supports both healing and health.

Chapter 12

Hemophilia: When the Body Can't Stop the Bleeding

Hemophilia is one of the most well-known blood disorders, characterized by a deficiency in certain clotting factors, which impairs the body's ability to form stable blood clots. This leads to the inability to stop bleeding after an injury or surgery, making even minor cuts or bruises potentially dangerous for individuals with this condition. Unlike some other bleeding disorders that stem from external factors, hemophilia is a genetic condition passed down from parent to child. For those living with hemophilia, the struggle to manage everyday life while preventing excessive bleeding can be both physically and emotionally challenging. This chapter explores the origins, symptoms, diagnosis, and management of hemophilia, shedding light on the realities of living with this chronic condition.

The Origins of Hemophilia: A Genetic Legacy

Hemophilia is a genetic disorder, meaning it is inherited from one or both parents. It is most commonly passed down through **X-linked recessive inheritance**, which explains why the condition predominantly affects males. The genes responsible for hemophilia are located on the **X chromosome**, and males, who only have one X chromosome, are at a higher risk of inheriting the condition. Females, who have two X chromosomes, are typically carriers of the gene and may pass it on to their offspring.

In hemophilia, a defect or mutation occurs in one of the genes that codes for clotting factors, proteins necessary for blood to clot properly. There are two main types of hemophilia:

1. **Hemophilia A**: This is the most common form of the condition and occurs due to a deficiency or absence of **factor VIII**, one of the proteins involved in the coagulation cascade. Factor VIII plays a critical role in helping platelets and other clotting factors form a stable clot. Without adequate factor VIII, the blood's ability to clot is compromised.
2. **Hemophilia B**: Also known as **Christmas disease**, hemophilia B is caused by a deficiency of **factor IX**. Like hemophilia A, it results in prolonged bleeding, but the treatment and management may differ slightly due to the different clotting factor involved.

Both types of hemophilia are inherited in a similar manner, with males affected most severely. Females can be carriers of the condition, which means they typically have one normal X chromosome and one mutated X chromosome. In some rare cases, females with hemophilia may experience mild symptoms, but this is unusual, as they typically have enough of the clotting factor from their unaffected X chromosome to compensate.

Symptoms of Hemophilia: A Bleeding Disorder with Lifelong Consequences

The hallmark symptom of hemophilia is **excessive bleeding**. People with hemophilia may experience difficulty stopping bleeding after even minor injuries, such as cuts or scrapes. Internal bleeding, especially into joints and muscles, is also common. These symptoms can range from mild to severe, depending on the degree of factor deficiency in the body.

The severity of hemophilia is typically categorized as follows:

- **Mild Hemophilia**: Individuals with mild hemophilia usually have a factor level of between 5% and 40% of normal. They may only experience bleeding problems after significant trauma or surgery. For instance, they might experience prolonged bleeding after dental work, surgery, or a major injury.
- **Moderate Hemophilia**: With moderate hemophilia, individuals have a factor level between 1% and 5% of normal. They are at a higher risk of spontaneous bleeding episodes, though these may occur less frequently than in severe cases.
- **Severe Hemophilia**: Severe hemophilia is characterized by a factor level of less than 1% of normal. People with severe hemophilia are at constant risk of spontaneous bleeding, even without obvious injuries. Bleeding episodes can occur inside the joints (known as **hemarthrosis**), muscles, and internal organs. These episodes are often painful and can lead to joint damage over time.

Common symptoms of hemophilia include:

- **Easy bruising**: Even minor bumps or pressure can lead to large bruises.
- **Prolonged bleeding after cuts**: This could be a small cut or a more significant injury.

- **Frequent nosebleeds**: People with hemophilia may have nosebleeds that last longer than normal or occur frequently without apparent cause.
- **Internal bleeding**: This includes bleeding into muscles, joints, or organs, which may occur spontaneously or after mild trauma.
- **Hemarthrosis**: Bleeding into the joints can cause swelling, pain, and limited movement. Over time, repeated bleeding into the joints can lead to joint deformities and long-term disability.

Diagnosing Hemophilia: Blood Tests and Family History

Diagnosing hemophilia involves a combination of clinical evaluation and laboratory tests. A physician will start by reviewing the patient's medical history, paying particular attention to any bleeding tendencies or family history of bleeding disorders. If hemophilia is suspected, a series of blood tests will be conducted to confirm the diagnosis.

The primary test for diagnosing hemophilia is the **activated partial thromboplastin time (aPTT)** test, which measures how long it takes for blood to clot. If the aPTT is prolonged, this suggests a clotting factor deficiency. Further tests will then be performed to measure the specific levels of clotting factors, particularly factor VIII or factor IX, depending on whether the patient is suspected of having hemophilia A or B.

In some cases, **genetic testing** may be used to identify mutations in the X chromosome, confirming the diagnosis and determining the specific mutation causing the condition. Genetic counseling is often recommended for families with a history of hemophilia to understand the inheritance pattern and assess the risk for future children.

Living with Hemophilia: Managing a Chronic Condition

Hemophilia is a lifelong condition that requires ongoing management to minimize the risk of bleeding and complications. The management of hemophilia typically involves:

1. **Factor Replacement Therapy**: The mainstay of treatment for hemophilia is the infusion of clotting factor concentrates to replace the deficient factor. This can be done on a regular basis to prevent spontaneous bleeding (prophylactic treatment) or as needed to stop a bleeding episode. Advances

in factor replacement therapy have greatly improved the quality of life for people with hemophilia, as these treatments can now be given at home.

2. **Desmopressin (DDAVP)**: For people with mild hemophilia A, desmopressin, a synthetic form of a hormone that helps release stored factor VIII, may be used to stimulate the body's own clotting factor production.

3. **Physical Therapy and Joint Care**: Repeated bleeding into joints (hemarthrosis) can cause joint damage and pain over time. Regular physical therapy helps maintain joint function and mobility. In some cases, surgery may be necessary to repair joint damage caused by frequent bleeds.

4. **Managing Bleeding Episodes**: People with hemophilia need to take precautions to avoid injury. This includes avoiding contact sports or wearing protective gear during physical activities. When bleeding does occur, prompt treatment with factor replacement is essential to prevent complications. In the case of severe internal bleeding, immediate medical attention is required to administer additional treatment.

5. **Regular Monitoring**: People with hemophilia must be closely monitored by healthcare providers. Regular blood tests are required to assess clotting factor levels and adjust treatment plans accordingly. Frequent check-ups are also needed to manage any complications, such as joint damage or inhibitor development (when the body develops antibodies against the clotting factor).

Challenges in Hemophilia Care: Access, Complications, and Emotional Impact

While advances in treatment have significantly improved the lives of people with hemophilia, challenges remain. Access to care is a major issue, particularly in low-income and developing regions, where factor replacement therapies may not be available or affordable. For individuals in such areas, the lack of treatment options can result in severe disability or even death from bleeding episodes.

Additionally, some individuals with hemophilia may develop **inhibitors**, which are antibodies that attack the infused clotting factors, making treatment less effective. This condition can make it more difficult to manage bleeding episodes, requiring alternative treatments such as immune tolerance therapy or bypass agents.

On an emotional level, living with hemophilia can take a toll on both individuals and their families. The constant fear of bleeding episodes, the burden of regular treatments, and the limitations placed on daily activities can lead to anxiety, depression, and social isolation. Support from healthcare providers, family, and community resources is crucial to helping people with hemophilia cope with these challenges and maintain a high quality of life.

Conclusion: Hope for the Future

While hemophilia is a lifelong condition with no cure, advances in treatment have made it possible for people with hemophilia to lead full, active lives. Gene therapy is an emerging treatment that holds promise for offering a more permanent solution to the disorder. By replacing or repairing the faulty gene responsible for hemophilia, gene therapy has the potential to significantly reduce or even eliminate the need for factor replacement therapy in the future.

The continued progress in hemophilia research and treatment provides hope for those affected by the condition. However, access to care, prevention of complications, and emotional support remain essential components of managing this genetic disorder. As society becomes more aware of the struggles faced by individuals with hemophilia, there is a growing movement to ensure better access to care, improved treatments, and a brighter future for all those living with hemophilia.

Chapter 13

The Spectrum of Hemophilia: Mild to Severe

Hemophilia is a complex genetic disorder, characterized by a deficiency or absence of certain clotting factors in the blood. The severity of hemophilia can vary significantly among affected individuals, ranging from mild to severe forms of the disease. This variation not only influences the severity of symptoms but also the approaches to diagnosis, treatment, and lifestyle adaptation. Understanding the spectrum of hemophilia is crucial for tailoring medical care and supporting individuals with this condition in leading active, fulfilling lives despite the challenges it presents. This chapter delves into the different levels of hemophilia, the diagnostic methods used to classify the severity, and how people with hemophilia adapt their lifestyles to manage their condition.

Mild Hemophilia: Living with Caution

Mild hemophilia is the least severe form of the disorder, typically characterized by clotting factor levels that range from 5% to 40% of normal levels. Individuals with mild hemophilia generally experience bleeding problems only after significant trauma or surgery. For instance, they may not notice any major symptoms following minor cuts or bruises but might experience prolonged bleeding after a major accident or medical procedure. This form of hemophilia is often not diagnosed until an injury or surgery occurs, making it somewhat difficult to detect early in life.

Symptoms and Diagnosis of Mild Hemophilia

People with mild hemophilia might not have frequent or spontaneous bleeding episodes. Instead, they may only experience unusual bleeding when faced with more substantial physical activity or surgical procedures. The first signs of hemophilia may include prolonged bleeding after a dental procedure, minor surgery, or a sports injury. For example, someone with mild hemophilia might experience excessive bleeding from a small cut or require medical intervention after a sprain or fracture. Hemorrhaging into the joints (hemarthrosis) or muscles may also occur under intense physical activity, although it's generally less frequent.

Diagnosing mild hemophilia often takes place later in life compared to more severe forms of the disorder. Doctors typically identify mild hemophilia through blood tests, such as the **activated partial thromboplastin time (aPTT)** test, which measures how long it takes for blood to clot. If the test is prolonged, further testing to assess the clotting factor levels is needed. If factor VIII (for hemophilia A) or factor IX (for hemophilia B) is found to be present at reduced levels, a diagnosis of mild hemophilia is confirmed.

Treatment and Lifestyle Adaptation for Mild Hemophilia

While individuals with mild hemophilia may not need daily factor replacement therapy, treatment is necessary when they experience significant bleeding events. People with mild hemophilia often receive clotting factor infusions on an as-needed basis (also called **on-demand treatment**) to address bleeding episodes or prevent bleeding during surgeries or dental procedures.

Because of the relatively mild nature of the condition, people with mild hemophilia are often able to lead relatively normal lives with some precautionary measures. For instance, they may avoid engaging in high-risk activities, such as contact sports, to reduce the likelihood of injury. However, with proper medical care, people with mild hemophilia can often participate in many physical activities, including low-impact exercise, with minimal risk.

Despite this, individuals with mild hemophilia must remain vigilant about their health and seek medical care when experiencing any signs of unusual bleeding. Regular check-ups with hematologists help monitor clotting factor levels and assess any changes that might require adjustments to treatment plans.

Moderate Hemophilia: The Balance Between Normal Life and Bleeding Risks

Moderate hemophilia is characterized by clotting factor levels between 1% and 5% of normal. Individuals with moderate hemophilia tend to experience more frequent bleeding episodes compared to those with the mild form, though these episodes are still less frequent than in individuals with severe hemophilia. Bleeding events may occur after moderate trauma or as a result of certain medical procedures, and spontaneous internal bleeding is possible, particularly in the joints and muscles.

Symptoms and Diagnosis of Moderate Hemophilia

Individuals with moderate hemophilia may bleed more often and with less provocation than those with mild hemophilia, but their bleeding episodes are generally not as severe as those in individuals with severe hemophilia. **Hemarthrosis**, or bleeding into the joints, is a common problem for people with moderate hemophilia, especially if the bleeding episodes are untreated or inadequately managed. Joint bleeding can lead to long-term joint damage, pain, and mobility issues if it occurs repeatedly.

Because people with moderate hemophilia experience more frequent symptoms, they are usually diagnosed earlier in life than individuals with the mild form. Diagnosis often occurs when a child is a toddler or early school-aged, especially after experiencing frequent bruising, nosebleeds, or prolonged bleeding from minor injuries.

Diagnosis follows similar steps as for mild hemophilia, with prolonged aPTT being followed by testing for specific clotting factor deficiencies. The factor level between 1% and 5% is indicative of moderate hemophilia. Early identification is important to implement treatment plans that can help reduce the frequency of bleeding episodes and prevent complications like joint damage.

Treatment and Lifestyle Adaptation for Moderate Hemophilia

People with moderate hemophilia typically require **prophylactic treatment**, which involves regular infusions of clotting factor to prevent bleeding episodes, especially as they approach certain milestones such as physical activities, dental procedures, or surgeries. The aim of prophylaxis is to maintain clotting factor levels at a sufficiently high level to avoid spontaneous bleeding. Some individuals with moderate hemophilia may also receive on-demand treatment if a bleeding episode occurs.

For individuals with moderate hemophilia, lifestyle adaptation revolves around avoiding activities that might cause excessive physical trauma, such as contact sports or heavy lifting. However, with proper medical support and treatment, many individuals with moderate hemophilia can engage in a wide variety of physical activities, including non-contact sports and exercise, which can help with joint health and overall physical well-being.

As people with moderate hemophilia grow older, they must also address concerns regarding long-term joint health, as repeated joint bleeds can lead to chronic pain, stiffness, and arthritis. Physical therapy and appropriate exercise regimens are often recommended to maintain joint mobility and prevent or slow the onset of joint damage.

Severe Hemophilia: Managing Life with Constant Vigilance

Severe hemophilia is the most serious form of the disorder, with clotting factor levels typically less than 1% of normal. Individuals with severe hemophilia face frequent spontaneous bleeding episodes, often without obvious triggers, and are at high risk of bleeding into joints (hemarthrosis) and internal organs. **Hemophilic arthropathy**, a condition involving joint damage due to repeated internal bleeding, is a common and disabling complication of severe hemophilia.

Symptoms and Diagnosis of Severe Hemophilia

Severe hemophilia presents at an early age, often in infancy or early childhood, and symptoms can be immediately apparent. Babies with severe hemophilia may experience excessive bruising from minor knocks or even spontaneous bleeding into the skin or mucous membranes. As the child grows and becomes more active, more significant bleeding episodes may occur, including joint bleeding, muscle bleeds, or even life-threatening internal bleeding.

Because the symptoms are severe and persistent, **early diagnosis** is critical. Babies and young children with severe hemophilia often experience repeated episodes of uncontrolled bleeding, which can require immediate medical intervention to prevent complications. Early diagnosis, typically confirmed through blood tests for clotting factor levels, is important for implementing aggressive treatment protocols to reduce the frequency and severity of bleeding events.

Treatment and Lifestyle Adaptation for Severe Hemophilia

For individuals with severe hemophilia, **prophylactic treatment** is essential. This involves regular infusions of clotting factors to maintain a target clotting factor level above a certain threshold, reducing the likelihood of spontaneous bleeding and allowing for better management of bleeding episodes when they do occur. Prophylactic treatment for severe hemophilia is generally more frequent, often several times per week, depending on the individual's needs.

Despite regular treatment, individuals with severe hemophilia must be vigilant about their lifestyle. Activities that carry a risk of injury, such as contact sports, high-impact exercises, or even certain recreational activities, are typically avoided. Protective gear may be necessary for engaging in low-risk activities, and safety measures are crucial when participating in everyday activities such as walking or playing.

Joint health is a significant concern for individuals with severe hemophilia, as frequent bleeding into the joints can lead to permanent damage, pain, and limited mobility. As a result, physical therapy is essential to help maintain joint function, and individuals with severe hemophilia may require surgical interventions or joint replacement surgery to manage long-term joint damage.

Adapting to the Spectrum of Hemophilia

Living with hemophilia, whether mild, moderate, or severe, requires a careful balance of treatment, prevention, and lifestyle adjustments. While those with mild hemophilia may experience few symptoms and lead relatively normal lives, those with severe hemophilia face constant vigilance and frequent medical interventions. Regardless of the severity, individuals with hemophilia share the common experience of managing a lifelong condition that impacts their physical health and emotional well-being.

Understanding the spectrum of hemophilia is critical for both medical professionals and individuals with the condition, as it guides the development of personalized treatment plans and lifestyle adjustments. Advances in medical treatments, including clotting factor replacement therapies, gene therapy, and joint protection strategies, continue to improve the quality of life for people with hemophilia, allowing them to live active, fulfilling lives while managing the risks associated with bleeding disorders.

The ability to adapt to the challenges posed by hemophilia, through a combination of medical care, safety precautions, and mental resilience, enables individuals to thrive in spite of the limitations imposed by their condition. And with continued research into better treatments and potential cures, the future holds promising possibilities for people living with hemophilia, regardless of the severity of their disease.

Chapter 14

Von Willebrand Disease: The Silent Bleeder

Von Willebrand Disease (VWD) is one of the most common inherited bleeding disorders, yet it remains widely underdiagnosed and often overlooked. Unlike hemophilia, which is more commonly associated with severe, noticeable bleeding episodes, VWD can present in ways that are less obvious, leading to a delayed diagnosis in many cases. This chapter provides an in-depth exploration of Von Willebrand Disease, a disorder that affects both men and women but is often misdiagnosed due to its subtle symptoms and overlapping characteristics with other bleeding conditions.

What is Von Willebrand Disease?

Von Willebrand Disease is a genetic bleeding disorder that affects the blood's ability to clot properly. This condition results from a deficiency or dysfunction of **von Willebrand factor (VWF)**, a crucial protein that helps platelets stick to the blood vessel wall and form blood clots. VWF also stabilizes **Factor VIII**, another important protein involved in the clotting process. Without adequate or functional VWF, the clotting cascade is disrupted, leading to an increased risk of bleeding.

Although VWD is a genetic disorder, it is often not diagnosed in infancy or childhood because its symptoms can be mild and easily dismissed as minor injuries or common issues. The disease can vary significantly in severity, from mild cases where the symptoms are so subtle that individuals may not even realize they have a bleeding disorder, to more severe cases with frequent, spontaneous bleeding events.

Types of Von Willebrand Disease

Von Willebrand Disease is classified into three main types: **Type 1, Type 2, and Type 3**. Each type has its own characteristics and varies in severity, but all types are linked to an abnormality in von Willebrand factor.

- **Type 1 VWD** is the mildest form and accounts for approximately 70-80% of all cases. People with Type 1 have reduced levels of von Willebrand factor, but still have enough of it to maintain some level of clotting ability.

Symptoms may include easy bruising, frequent nosebleeds, heavy menstrual bleeding, or mild bleeding after dental procedures or minor surgery. Because the symptoms are not as severe as those seen in Type 2 or Type 3, many individuals may go undiagnosed or misdiagnosed for years.

- **Type 2 VWD** is a more moderate form of the disease, where the von Willebrand factor is either qualitatively defective or dysfunctional. This type is divided into four subtypes (2A, 2B, 2M, and 2N), each with its own pattern of dysfunction in the VWF protein. People with Type 2 VWD may experience more frequent bleeding episodes, such as joint bleeds, and might also experience an increased tendency to bleed even from minor injuries.
- **Type 3 VWD** is the most severe form of the disorder, and it is much rarer than Type 1 or Type 2. In Type 3 VWD, individuals have little or no von Willebrand factor, which leads to a significantly higher risk of spontaneous bleeding episodes, such as deep bruising, internal bleeding, or bleeding into the joints and muscles (hemarthrosis). This form of VWD is often diagnosed in childhood due to the severity of symptoms, and it may require intensive treatment to manage the bleeding risks.

Symptoms of Von Willebrand Disease

The symptoms of Von Willebrand Disease can range from mild to severe, depending on the type of the disorder and the individual's clotting factor levels. Some common signs and symptoms include:

- **Easy Bruising:** Individuals with VWD may notice that they bruise more easily than others, often from minor bumps or injuries.
- **Frequent Nosebleeds:** Recurrent nosebleeds that are difficult to stop are a hallmark symptom of VWD, especially in younger children.
- **Heavy Menstrual Bleeding:** Women with VWD often experience unusually heavy or prolonged menstrual periods, a condition known as **menorrhagia**. In some cases, they may pass large blood clots or experience prolonged bleeding after childbirth or a miscarriage.
- **Prolonged Bleeding from Cuts or Surgery:** Even minor cuts or surgical procedures, such as a tooth extraction, may cause prolonged bleeding in individuals with VWD.
- **Joint and Muscle Bleeding:** In more severe cases of VWD (Type 2 and Type 3), bleeding into the joints or muscles can occur, leading to pain, swelling, and long-term damage to the joints.

- **Gastrointestinal Bleeding:** In some individuals, VWD can lead to bleeding in the digestive tract, which may result in black, tarry stools or other symptoms of internal bleeding.

One of the reasons VWD is often not immediately diagnosed is that its symptoms can resemble those of other more common bleeding disorders, like platelet dysfunction or even the bleeding tendency observed in people taking certain medications like aspirin. Because of the wide spectrum of symptoms and severity, VWD can sometimes be misinterpreted as a mild form of a different condition, leading to delays in diagnosis and treatment.

Diagnosing Von Willebrand Disease

Diagnosing Von Willebrand Disease can be complex due to the overlap of its symptoms with other bleeding disorders, as well as the variation in severity across the three types. A thorough medical history is essential, especially in identifying family members who may also have a history of bleeding problems. Blood tests play a key role in diagnosing VWD and determining the type and severity of the disorder.

Some of the most common tests used to diagnose Von Willebrand Disease include:

- **von Willebrand Factor Antigen (VWF**

   ): This test measures the amount of von Willebrand factor present in the blood. Low levels suggest a possible diagnosis of VWD.

- **Ristocetin Cofactor Activity:** This test assesses the functionality of the von Willebrand factor, specifically how well it interacts with platelets. Abnormal results can help identify different subtypes of VWD.
- **Factor VIII Activity:** Since von Willebrand factor stabilizes Factor VIII, people with VWD may have reduced levels of Factor VIII. This test is used to assess the clotting activity of Factor VIII in the blood.
- **VWF Multimers:** This test examines the size and structure of the von Willebrand factor molecules. In Type 2 VWD, the von Willebrand factor may be abnormal in size or structure, which can be identified with this test.
- **Platelet Function Tests:** These tests evaluate how well platelets are able to form clots in the blood. Abnormal results may indicate platelet dysfunction, which can be a feature of some types of VWD.

Once diagnosed, further testing can determine the specific subtype of VWD, which is essential for tailoring treatment and management strategies.

Treating Von Willebrand Disease

The treatment of Von Willebrand Disease is aimed at controlling bleeding episodes and preventing complications. The approach to treatment will depend on the type and severity of the disease, as well as the individual's unique bleeding tendencies.

Desmopressin (DDAVP)

For individuals with **Type 1 VWD**, desmopressin (DDAVP) may be used to increase the release of von Willebrand factor from the body's stores. This can help temporarily raise von Willebrand factor levels and reduce the likelihood of bleeding during minor bleeding episodes or surgical procedures. DDAVP can be administered as an injection or nasal spray and is often effective in managing mild to moderate symptoms of the disease.

Clotting Factor Concentrates

For individuals with **Type 2 or Type 3 VWD**, treatment typically involves clotting factor concentrates that contain von Willebrand factor and factor VIII. These concentrates are administered intravenously to raise the levels of these clotting factors in the blood and prevent bleeding episodes. People with Type 3 VWD may require more frequent and higher doses of clotting factor concentrates, while those with Type 2 may require specific concentrates based on their subtype.

Antifibrinolytic Drugs

For some people with VWD, particularly those who experience heavy menstrual bleeding or excessive bleeding after dental procedures, **antifibrinolytic drugs** may be used to help stabilize blood clots and prevent them from breaking down prematurely. These medications can be taken orally or applied topically.

Hormonal Treatments

For women with **heavy menstrual bleeding** associated with VWD, hormonal treatments, such as birth control pills, intrauterine devices (IUDs), or hormone injections, may be recommended to help regulate menstrual cycles and reduce bleeding.

Surgical Interventions

In cases of severe bleeding or joint damage, surgical intervention may be necessary. People with VWD who experience **joint bleeds** or significant internal bleeding may require procedures to stop the bleeding or repair damaged tissues. Joint replacement surgery may also be an option for those with severe hemarthrosis, although this is typically considered after other treatment options have been exhausted.

Living with Von Willebrand Disease

Living with Von Willebrand Disease requires ongoing management and care to prevent bleeding episodes and address potential complications. People with VWD must work closely with their healthcare team to monitor bleeding tendencies, manage treatment plans, and take steps to avoid situations that may trigger excessive bleeding, such as taking precautions during sports or activities that pose a higher risk of injury.

Because VWD is a genetic disorder, it's important for individuals with the condition to understand its inheritance patterns, especially when planning families. Genetic counseling can help families better understand their risks and make informed decisions.

Conclusion

Von Willebrand Disease is a disorder that can silently impact a person's life, often without clear or immediate symptoms. While many people live with mild forms of the disease without even realizing it, others may face severe and life-threatening bleeding complications. Early diagnosis, accurate classification of the type of VWD, and appropriate treatment strategies are crucial for managing the disorder and improving the quality of life for those affected. Despite its subtle nature, Von Willebrand Disease is a treatable condition, and with ongoing medical advancements, individuals with VWD can lead fulfilling, active lives.

Chapter 15

Living with Hemophilia: Coping and Adaptation

Hemophilia is a rare and often misunderstood condition, one that forces individuals to adapt their lives in ways that most of us never imagine. Living with hemophilia means living with the constant challenge of managing a bleeding disorder that can affect every part of life. While medical advances have improved the prognosis for many people living with hemophilia, the psychological and social impacts are profound. For those living with the condition, the struggle to maintain a sense of normalcy in their daily routines is a lifelong journey of resilience and adaptation.

In this chapter, we'll delve into personal stories from individuals living with hemophilia, exploring how they cope with the challenges posed by the condition. From navigating school and social activities as children to managing work and family life as adults, we will look at how people with hemophilia confront their fears, find strength, and push through the limitations imposed by their disease.

The Early Years: Navigating Childhood with Hemophilia

For many children diagnosed with hemophilia, the early years are marked by uncertainty and the heightened vigilance of their families. Hemophilia is often diagnosed in infancy, when parents may notice unusual bleeding or bruising after minor injuries or medical procedures. From the outset, these families must come to terms with a new reality: that their child's body cannot stop bleeding in the same way that others can. This can be a difficult adjustment, especially for parents who must monitor every bump and bruise their child sustains.

James's Story: Coping with the Fear of Injury

James, a 12-year-old boy diagnosed with hemophilia at the age of 2, has known about his condition for as long as he can remember. His mother, Emily, recounts the fear they both felt when he was diagnosed: "We didn't know what to expect. I remember being terrified when he started crawling, because every fall seemed like it could be life-threatening. But over time, we learned how to manage his condition."

James's life, like many other children with hemophilia, has been shaped by a series of precautions. He is prohibited from participating in contact sports, and even physical activities like biking or skateboarding are undertaken with great caution. At school, James wears protective gear when playing sports, and his teachers are trained to recognize the signs of a bleed. Despite these challenges, James has adapted to his condition with the help of his family, friends, and a strong medical team. "I can't do everything other kids can do, but I can still play sports and hang out with my friends. I just have to be careful and listen to my body."

Although James lives with the limitations of his condition, he refuses to let hemophilia define his life. His parents have made it a priority to expose him to a variety of activities, fostering his confidence in the process. However, it's clear that for James and his family, living with hemophilia has been a balancing act between keeping him safe and allowing him the freedom to be a child.

Teenage Years: Identity, Independence, and Risk

As children with hemophilia grow older, the challenges evolve. Adolescence brings the desire for independence, but it also introduces more complicated social dynamics and the inevitable exposure to risks, such as driving, partying, and taking part in physical activities outside of structured environments. The teenage years are often the most difficult time for many people with hemophilia, as they navigate not only the physical limitations imposed by their condition but also the emotional and psychological aspects of living with a chronic illness.

Sophia's Story: Finding Balance Between Normalcy and Caution

Sophia, now 17, has lived with hemophilia since birth. Growing up, she had the usual bumps and bruises that every child experiences, but her parents always ensured that she had access to medical care and appropriate treatments when needed. As a teenager, however, Sophia began to wrestle with her condition in ways she hadn't before. "When I hit my teenage years, I just wanted to be like everyone else. I wanted to go to parties and try things that my friends were doing, but I was always scared of bleeding," she says.

Sophia's struggle to find balance between normal teen experiences and the constraints of hemophilia was intense. She remembers, "There were times when I wanted to just let go and enjoy life. But I had to remind myself that I couldn't do things like go rock climbing or play football without really thinking about the consequences."

For Sophia, hemophilia is both an invisible and highly visible condition. In social settings, she often feels isolated because people can't immediately see the challenges she faces. "I remember one time at a party when I fell and scraped my knee, and everyone was like, 'Oh, that's just a small cut.' But I knew the implications of that small injury could be huge if I wasn't careful."

Sophia learned that self-advocacy was crucial. "I had to get comfortable telling people about my condition—especially when I was in new situations, like at parties or sleepovers. I started carrying a medical alert bracelet, and I would remind my friends and their parents about my hemophilia. It wasn't easy, but it helped me feel less worried."

For Sophia, the teenage years were a time of self-discovery, resilience, and self-care. She gradually learned how to make responsible choices while still embracing independence. She acknowledges, "It's a delicate balance, but it's something I've had to learn over time."

Adulthood: Embracing Responsibility and Leading a Full Life

As individuals with hemophilia transition into adulthood, the focus shifts from childhood precautions to career, relationships, and long-term health management. The decision-making process becomes even more complicated, as adults with hemophilia must manage their condition while striving for autonomy and pursuing their life goals.

Ethan's Story: Thriving in the Workplace and in Family Life

Ethan, 35, was diagnosed with hemophilia A at the age of 4. Today, he is married with two children and works as an architect in a busy firm. Living with hemophilia has never been easy for Ethan, but he's learned how to live a fulfilling life. "When I was younger, I wasn't sure if I'd ever be able to have a normal job or start a family. But now, I realize that my condition doesn't have to hold me back. I just have to be smart about how I live my life."

Ethan is open about his condition at work and takes steps to ensure his colleagues understand the importance of keeping his medical needs in mind. "I've had to have several conversations with my employer and coworkers about what hemophilia is and what to do if something happens. Luckily, my workplace has been really supportive. I also take time off when I need to rest or recover from bleeds, but overall, I've learned to manage my work and health," he shares.

One of the most significant challenges Ethan faces is the physical strain of his condition. Like many adults with hemophilia, Ethan has developed arthritis in his joints due to the long-term effects of joint bleeds. He undergoes regular physiotherapy and maintains a careful exercise routine to help manage his pain. "Staying active is important, but I have to be cautious. I can't play full-contact sports anymore, but I enjoy swimming and light weightlifting. The key is consistency and knowing my limits," he explains.

Family life also presents unique challenges. Raising two young children while managing hemophilia has required Ethan and his wife, Lisa, to stay vigilant. "We had to be proactive about our children's health from the moment they were born. Luckily, neither of them has hemophilia, but we made sure they understood what hemophilia is and how they can help in emergencies," he says. For Ethan and his family, the priority is maintaining a balance between everyday life and his health, and they work together to ensure that their household runs smoothly despite the complexities of hemophilia.

Mental and Emotional Resilience: Coping with the Emotional Toll

In addition to the physical challenges of hemophilia, living with a bleeding disorder also takes a psychological toll. People with hemophilia often struggle with anxiety, stress, and the emotional burden of managing a chronic illness. Fear of bleeding episodes, concerns about the future, and feelings of isolation are common struggles for many.

Charlotte's Story: Finding Strength in Therapy and Support Groups

Charlotte, 28, was diagnosed with hemophilia at age 3. Throughout her life, she has experienced both physical pain and emotional turmoil, particularly when dealing with frequent joint bleeds. "I used to be afraid to leave the house because I was always scared something would happen," Charlotte admits. "I would avoid going out with friends or traveling, because I didn't want to risk bleeding in an unfamiliar place."

Over time, Charlotte sought therapy to help manage her anxiety. "Talking about hemophilia and how it impacts my mental health was life-changing. I realized that I didn't have to go through it alone," she says. Charlotte also found strength in support groups, where she could connect with others who understood her struggles. "Being part of a community of people who get it has been incredibly empowering."

Through therapy and support from her peers, Charlotte has learned how to better manage her emotions. She practices mindfulness and uses stress-reduction techniques, which help her remain calm during times of uncertainty. "Hemophilia will always be a part of my life, but it doesn't have to control me. I'm learning how to live with it, not be defined by it," Charlotte reflects.

Conclusion: Resilience and Empowerment

Living with hemophilia is undeniably challenging, but those who face this condition find ways to thrive despite it. Whether it's coping with the limitations during childhood, navigating the pressures of adolescence, or adapting to adulthood, individuals with hemophilia demonstrate extraordinary resilience and strength. They refuse to be defined by their condition, and through a combination of medical care, mental fortitude, and supportive communities, they lead lives full of accomplishment, connection, and meaning. As hemophilia awareness and treatments continue to improve, so too will the lives of those living with the disorder, offering hope for a future where they can live their fullest, healthiest lives.

Chapter 16

Anticoagulants: Managing the Risks of Clotting and Bleeding

Anticoagulants, often referred to as blood-thinning medications, play a critical role in the management of various blood clotting disorders. These medications work by reducing the blood's ability to form clots, thus helping prevent dangerous conditions such as deep vein thrombosis (DVT), pulmonary embolism, and stroke. While they can be lifesaving for many individuals, anticoagulants also carry inherent risks of bleeding, which makes their management a delicate balancing act for both patients and healthcare providers.

This chapter will explore the role of anticoagulants in treating blood clotting disorders, the different types available, their mechanisms of action, potential side effects, and how individuals on anticoagulants can navigate the delicate balance between preventing clots and avoiding excessive bleeding.

The Importance of Blood Clotting and the Need for Anticoagulants

Before delving into anticoagulants specifically, it's essential to understand why blood clotting is so important. Blood clotting is a natural response of the body to injury. When a blood vessel is damaged, the body triggers a process known as coagulation, where platelets clump together to form a clot that plugs the wound, preventing excessive blood loss. At the same time, various proteins in the blood, known as clotting factors, work to solidify and stabilize the clot, creating a protective barrier over the damaged area.

However, blood clotting can sometimes occur unnecessarily, leading to harmful conditions. When clots form inappropriately, without injury or in an area where the clot might travel to vital organs, they can cause severe complications. For example, clots in the deep veins of the legs can travel to the lungs, causing a pulmonary embolism (PE), a potentially fatal condition. Similarly, clots in the brain can lead to strokes, which may cause permanent neurological damage. Anticoagulants work to prevent these types of complications by reducing the clotting ability of the blood.

Types of Anticoagulants

There are several types of anticoagulants, each working in different ways to prevent blood clot formation. The primary categories include direct oral anticoagulants (DOACs), vitamin K antagonists (such as warfarin), and heparins, which are often administered in hospital settings.

1. Warfarin (Coumadin)

Warfarin, one of the oldest and most widely used anticoagulants, is a vitamin K antagonist. It works by inhibiting the action of vitamin K, which is necessary for the production of clotting factors. By interfering with vitamin K's role, warfarin reduces the production of clotting factors, making it harder for blood to form clots.

Warfarin has been a cornerstone in the treatment and prevention of conditions like atrial fibrillation (a common cause of stroke), deep vein thrombosis (DVT), and pulmonary embolism (PE). Despite its effectiveness, warfarin requires close monitoring, typically through regular blood tests that measure the International Normalized Ratio (INR). The INR tests the time it takes for blood to clot and ensures that the anticoagulant effect of warfarin remains within a therapeutic range, minimizing the risk of both clotting and bleeding.

However, warfarin's effectiveness can be influenced by various factors, including diet (specifically the intake of foods rich in vitamin K), other medications, and even lifestyle changes. This requires patients to be vigilant about maintaining a consistent diet and adhering to regular blood testing to ensure they stay within the prescribed therapeutic range.

2. Direct Oral Anticoagulants (DOACs)

Direct oral anticoagulants (DOACs) are a newer class of anticoagulants that offer several advantages over warfarin. The most commonly used DOACs include **dabigatran (Pradaxa)**, **rivaroxaban (Xarelto)**, **apixaban (Eliquis)**, and **edoxaban (Savaysa)**. These medications work by directly inhibiting specific clotting factors, such as factor Xa or thrombin (factor IIa), which play essential roles in the coagulation process.

One of the key benefits of DOACs over warfarin is that they do not require routine blood monitoring. The therapeutic effect of DOACs is more predictable, allowing patients to maintain a more consistent dosing regimen without the need for frequent lab tests. DOACs are also less influenced by food interactions, making them easier to incorporate into daily life.

Despite these benefits, DOACs are not without risks. They are still relatively new compared to warfarin, which has a long history of use. Additionally, there are no widely available antidotes for some DOACs, meaning that in cases of severe bleeding, managing these complications can be more challenging. However, there have been significant advancements in the development of reversal agents for some DOACs, such as **idarucizumab** for dabigatran, which provide added safety in emergency situations.

3. Heparins

Heparins are a class of anticoagulants commonly used in hospital settings, particularly for patients who need immediate anticoagulation therapy. **Unfractionated heparin (UFH)** and **low molecular weight heparin (LMWH)** are the two main types of heparins, and both act by inhibiting clotting factors to prevent blood from clotting excessively.

Unfractionated heparin is typically administered intravenously and requires frequent blood monitoring to adjust the dose as needed. It is often used in acute situations, such as during a heart attack or major surgery. Low molecular weight heparin, on the other hand, can be injected subcutaneously and is more predictable, requiring less frequent monitoring. It is often used for long-term prevention of blood clots, particularly in patients with DVT, PE, or those undergoing hip or knee replacement surgery.

Heparin, like warfarin, can lead to complications such as bleeding, which is why it is typically used in controlled hospital settings where the patient's condition can be closely monitored.

The Risks and Benefits of Anticoagulants

While anticoagulants are crucial for preventing life-threatening clots, they also pose a significant risk of bleeding. This paradox—the risk of excessive bleeding versus the risk of dangerous clot formation—makes the use of anticoagulants a complex decision that requires careful monitoring.

Bleeding Risks

The primary concern when using anticoagulants is the increased risk of bleeding. This can range from minor bleeding, such as nosebleeds or bruising, to more severe complications, including gastrointestinal bleeding, brain hemorrhages, or life-threatening internal bleeding. For patients on anticoagulants, even a minor fall or injury can become a major medical emergency.

Bleeding complications can be especially dangerous in individuals who are older or have other health conditions that increase the risk of bleeding, such as liver disease or a history of gastrointestinal ulcers. Monitoring is crucial, particularly for patients on warfarin, who require regular blood tests to ensure their clotting levels remain within a safe range. Similarly, for those on DOACs, while monitoring is not required, it's still important to be vigilant about symptoms of bleeding and to communicate regularly with healthcare providers.

Clotting Risks

On the flip side, failing to use anticoagulants when they are needed can increase the risk of clot formation. In people with conditions like atrial fibrillation, the blood flow through the heart can become irregular, leading to the formation of clots that can travel to the brain and cause a stroke. In these cases, anticoagulants are used not only to prevent clots from forming but also to reduce the risk of life-threatening complications.

For individuals with conditions like deep vein thrombosis (DVT), anticoagulants are essential to prevent clots from traveling to the lungs, where they can cause a pulmonary embolism. Without anticoagulation therapy, these clots would likely grow larger and more dangerous.

Living with Anticoagulants: Patient Management and Lifestyle

For people prescribed anticoagulants, life often involves a careful balancing act between preventing clotting and minimizing the risk of bleeding. Patients must be diligent about following their prescribed treatment plan, taking the medication as directed, and regularly visiting healthcare providers to monitor their condition. Additionally, lifestyle changes may be necessary to ensure safety.

Patients on anticoagulants are generally advised to avoid activities that pose a high risk of injury, such as contact sports or dangerous physical activities. They may also be asked to modify their diet to avoid foods that could interfere with their medication. For example, individuals on warfarin are encouraged to maintain a consistent intake of vitamin K, which can affect how the medication works.

Some patients may also need to take additional precautions, such as using softer toothbrushes or wearing medical alert bracelets, to ensure they are prepared for potential bleeding episodes.

The Future of Anticoagulant Therapy

The field of anticoagulation therapy continues to evolve, with ongoing research focused on improving the safety and efficacy of blood-thinning medications. New anticoagulants are being developed with more predictable effects, fewer side effects, and better options for reversing bleeding in emergencies. As these medications become more advanced, they hold the potential to make blood clot management safer and more effective for those living with clotting disorders.

In conclusion, anticoagulants are essential tools in the fight against blood clotting disorders, helping to reduce the risk of life-threatening conditions like stroke, DVT, and PE. However, their use comes with risks, and patients must work closely with their healthcare providers to ensure the best possible outcomes. By understanding the types of anticoagulants available, their mechanisms of action, and how to manage their risks, patients can lead healthier, more balanced lives while minimizing the potential dangers associated with clotting and bleeding disorders.

Chapter 17

Sickle Cell Disease: A Legacy of Mutation

Sickle cell disease (SCD), a genetic blood disorder, represents one of the most profound and widespread medical conditions affecting millions of people around the world. This inherited disorder primarily impacts the shape and function of red blood cells, leading to a cascade of symptoms that can profoundly affect an individual's health, quality of life, and even life expectancy. Though much is known about the disease, its origins, challenges, and continued impact remain a critical focus for medical researchers, health practitioners, and families.

In this chapter, we will explore the genetic basis of sickle cell disease, how it is inherited, its prevalence around the globe, the far-reaching effects it has on families, and the ongoing battle for better treatments. As we unravel the details of this disease, we will also highlight the resilience of those living with sickle cell disease, and the support systems that help manage its complexities.

The Genetic Basis of Sickle Cell Disease

Sickle cell disease is caused by a mutation in the gene that encodes for hemoglobin, the protein in red blood cells responsible for transporting oxygen throughout the body. Hemoglobin is made up of four subunits, two of which are called alpha-globin chains, and two are called beta-globin chains. In healthy individuals, the beta-globin chains are made from a specific sequence of amino acids that form normal hemoglobin (HbA).

However, in people with sickle cell disease, the mutation in the beta-globin gene results in the production of abnormal hemoglobin known as **hemoglobin S (HbS)**. This mutated hemoglobin causes red blood cells to take on an unusual, crescent or sickle-like shape, rather than their normal round, flexible shape. These sickle-shaped cells are stiff and sticky, and they can block blood flow through small blood vessels, leading to painful episodes and potentially causing organ damage.

The mutation that causes sickle cell disease is inherited in an **autosomal recessive pattern**, meaning that a person must inherit two copies of the mutated gene—one from each parent—to develop the disease. Individuals who inherit one normal gene and one mutated gene are referred to as **sickle cell trait** carriers.

While they typically do not experience the symptoms of sickle cell disease, they can pass the mutated gene on to their children.

This inheritance pattern explains the prevalence of sickle cell disease in certain populations, particularly those with African, Mediterranean, Middle Eastern, and Indian ancestry. The mutation confers a survival advantage against malaria, which is why the disease is more common in areas where malaria is endemic. The sickle cell trait can help individuals survive malaria, which is why the gene mutation persists in these populations despite its detrimental effects when two copies of the gene are inherited.

Prevalence of Sickle Cell Disease

Sickle cell disease affects millions of people worldwide, with an estimated **300,000 babies** born each year with severe forms of the disease. It is particularly prevalent in sub-Saharan Africa, where an estimated **1 in 4 people** carry the sickle cell trait. In the United States, approximately **100,000 individuals** are living with sickle cell disease, the majority of whom are of African descent, although the disease also affects individuals from other ethnic backgrounds, including Hispanic, Mediterranean, and Middle Eastern populations.

In the United States, sickle cell disease is most commonly diagnosed in newborns through routine newborn screening programs, which have significantly improved early diagnosis and care. Screening programs allow for the early identification of affected infants, ensuring that they receive timely treatments and interventions to manage symptoms and improve quality of life.

Sickle cell disease is also common in many countries in sub-Saharan Africa, where the disease places a heavy burden on healthcare systems. Limited access to healthcare and treatment options in these regions contributes to higher mortality rates associated with sickle cell disease. Advances in medical care and treatments are gradually improving survival rates, but the disease remains a major health challenge.

Pathophysiology of Sickle Cell Disease

The hallmark feature of sickle cell disease is the sickling of red blood cells under low oxygen conditions. In normal circumstances, red blood cells are flexible and can travel through small blood vessels to deliver oxygen to tissues. However, the presence of hemoglobin S in red blood cells causes them to change shape, particularly when oxygen levels in the blood decrease. This sickling is most apparent during physical exertion, illness, or dehydration—conditions where the oxygen demands of the body are increased.

Once sickled, the red blood cells lose their ability to flow smoothly through the blood vessels. They become rigid, sticky, and more prone to clumping together, which can block blood flow. This leads to a range of complications, including:

- **Pain crises (vaso-occlusive crises)**: These occur when sickled cells block blood flow, causing sudden and severe pain in the chest, abdomen, bones, and joints. Pain crises are a hallmark symptom of sickle cell disease and can last from hours to days. They can be triggered by infection, dehydration, cold temperatures, or stress.
- **Anemia**: The sickle-shaped red blood cells are fragile and have a shorter lifespan than normal red blood cells. While healthy red blood cells live for about 120 days, sickle cells only survive for 10-20 days. This leads to chronic anemia, where the body does not have enough healthy red blood cells to carry oxygen to tissues.
- **Organ damage**: Over time, the blockages in blood vessels can cause damage to vital organs, including the kidneys, liver, spleen, and heart. In particular, the spleen, which helps filter bacteria from the blood, can become damaged in early childhood, leaving individuals with sickle cell disease more vulnerable to infections.
- **Stroke**: The blockage of blood flow to the brain can result in a stroke, which is one of the most serious complications of sickle cell disease. Children with sickle cell disease are at particular risk for stroke, which can cause lifelong neurological deficits.
- **Infections**: People with sickle cell disease have a weakened immune system, and the spleen is particularly affected by the disease. As a result, they are more prone to infections caused by bacteria, especially pneumococcus. Vaccination and regular antibiotic prophylaxis are essential for infection prevention.

Impact on Families and Communities

Sickle cell disease has a profound impact not only on individuals but also on their families and communities. The disease's chronic nature means that affected individuals often require lifelong medical care, which can be expensive and emotionally taxing for families. Parents of children with sickle cell disease often become experts in managing their child's symptoms, coordinating medical care, and navigating the challenges of school and social activities.

The burden of sickle cell disease on families can be both physical and emotional. Parents must cope with frequent hospital visits, pain crises, and the stress of managing the disease day to day. For children with the disease, the limitations placed on their activities due to pain or fatigue can affect their ability to engage in typical childhood experiences like playing sports or participating in school events.

The disease also has financial implications. Hospital stays, medications, blood transfusions, and regular check-ups can become costly, especially in regions with limited healthcare resources. For families in low-income or resource-poor areas, the financial and logistical challenges of managing sickle cell disease can be overwhelming.

In many cultures, there is a strong sense of community support that helps families manage the challenges of sickle cell disease. Support groups, patient advocacy organizations, and peer networks provide valuable emotional and practical assistance to families affected by sickle cell disease. These communities offer a space for individuals and families to share experiences, learn about new treatments, and access resources that can improve their lives.

Current Treatments and Management

While there is no universal cure for sickle cell disease, treatments have advanced considerably over the years, improving both quality of life and life expectancy for many individuals living with the disease. The main goals of treatment are to manage symptoms, prevent complications, and improve overall health.

Pain Management

Pain crises, or vaso-occlusive crises, are one of the most common and distressing symptoms of sickle cell disease. Treatment often involves pain relief strategies, which may include over-the-counter medications, stronger prescription pain relievers (such as opioids), and intravenous fluids to help prevent dehydration and manage pain during a crisis. Some individuals may require hospitalization during severe pain episodes.

Blood Transfusions

Regular blood transfusions are a common treatment for individuals with sickle cell disease, particularly those who experience severe anemia or who are at high risk for stroke. Transfusions can help reduce the number of sickle cells in the bloodstream, thus improving oxygen delivery and reducing the risk of complications. However, long-term transfusions carry risks, including iron overload, which can damage organs if not managed properly.

Hydroxyurea

Hydroxyurea is a medication that can reduce the frequency of pain crises and the need for blood transfusions by increasing the production of fetal hemoglobin (HbF), a type of hemoglobin that does not sickle. It is one of the few drugs that has been shown to reduce the severity of sickle cell disease symptoms and is often used for individuals with moderate to severe disease.

Bone Marrow and Stem Cell Transplantation

A bone marrow or stem cell transplant is currently the only potential cure for sickle cell disease. This procedure involves replacing the patient's bone marrow with that of a healthy donor, which can lead to the production of normal red blood cells. While successful transplants have been performed, this treatment is not suitable for everyone, and it carries significant risks, including graft-versus-host disease (GVHD) and rejection.

The Road Ahead: Hope for the Future

While sickle cell disease remains a lifelong challenge for many, ongoing research offers hope for the future. Advances in gene therapy and other cutting-edge treatments hold the potential for a cure or more effective management of the disease. Researchers are exploring ways to repair the defective hemoglobin gene, which could lead to a functional cure for individuals with sickle cell disease.

As awareness of sickle cell disease continues to grow and as research efforts intensify, the hope is that future generations will have access to better treatments and, ultimately, a cure. In the meantime, individuals and families affected by sickle cell disease continue to demonstrate incredible resilience and strength as they cope with the challenges of the disorder.

Sickle cell disease is more than just a medical condition; it is a deeply embedded part of the cultural and familial fabric for many around the world. Through increased research, better education, and more accessible healthcare, we can continue to improve the lives of those living with this challenging condition.

Chapter 18

The Crisis of Sickle Cell: Pain, Stroke, and Organ Damage

Sickle cell disease (SCD) is a chronic and potentially life-threatening condition, not only because of its genetic origins but also due to the numerous complications that arise from its progression. The hallmark of SCD is the sickling of red blood cells, which causes them to become rigid, sticky, and prone to blocking blood flow in small vessels. This impaired circulation leads to a wide array of complications, many of which can dramatically impact the health and quality of life of individuals living with the disease. These complications include excruciating pain crises, strokes, and organ damage, which are all too common in people with SCD. While medical treatments have made strides in alleviating some of these symptoms, the effects of SCD continue to present significant challenges.

In this chapter, we will explore the various complications of sickle cell disease, their underlying causes, and how patients manage these challenges in their daily lives. We will examine the physiological mechanisms behind pain crises, the risk of strokes, the organs affected by the disease, and the steps that individuals with SCD take to manage their health.

Pain Crises: The Heart of Sickle Cell Disease

Pain is arguably the most common and debilitating complication of sickle cell disease. The term "pain crisis" or **vaso-occlusive crisis (VOC)** describes the episodes when sickle-shaped red blood cells block blood flow in small blood vessels, causing a cascade of painful events. During these crises, blood flow to specific areas of the body becomes restricted, leading to oxygen deprivation in tissues and severe, localized pain.

The Mechanism Behind Pain Crises

Pain crises typically occur when sickle cells become more rigid and stick together under conditions of low oxygen, dehydration, or cold. The blocked blood vessels cause pain and inflammation in the affected area. The most common sites of pain are the bones, joints, chest, and abdomen. For children, VOCs are often seen in the long bones of the limbs, causing excruciating pain and difficulty with mobility. Adults often experience severe pain in their chest, bones, or back, which can incapacitate them for hours or even days.

A pain crisis can last anywhere from a few hours to several days. The pain is often described as sharp, stabbing, or throbbing, and its intensity can vary. These episodes are unpredictable, and individuals with SCD may go months without a crisis, only to experience one triggered by an infection, dehydration, or other stressors on the body. Frequent pain episodes are known to negatively affect a person's mental health, contributing to feelings of frustration, anxiety, and depression.

Management of Pain Crises

Management of pain crises is a central aspect of sickle cell disease treatment. The approach to pain management typically involves:

- **Hydration**: Maintaining adequate hydration is critical, as dehydration can exacerbate sickling and increase the severity of pain crises. Oral fluids are recommended, and in severe cases, intravenous fluids may be administered to prevent dehydration and improve circulation.
- **Pain Medications**: The first line of treatment for pain during a VOC is usually over-the-counter pain relievers such as acetaminophen or ibuprofen. For more severe pain, stronger medications, such as opioid painkillers, may be prescribed. Hospitals may administer intravenous pain relief when crises are particularly severe.
- **Oxygen Therapy**: In some cases, supplemental oxygen may be used to increase oxygen delivery to the tissues and help relieve pain during a crisis. This is particularly helpful in cases where the pain is due to a lack of oxygen in the blood.
- **Physical Rest**: Limiting physical activity during a crisis allows the body to focus on recovery and helps prevent further strain on the already compromised circulatory system.

While pain management strategies are essential in the acute treatment of VOCs, the challenge lies in preventing frequent crises. Medications such as **hydroxyurea** have been shown to reduce the frequency of pain crises by stimulating the production of fetal hemoglobin (HbF), a type of hemoglobin that does not sickle.

Stroke: A Life-Threatening Complication

Stroke is one of the most severe complications associated with sickle cell disease. It occurs when the blood flow to the brain is interrupted, either due to blood vessels being blocked by sickle cells or because of hemorrhage caused by fragile blood vessels. People with sickle cell disease are at increased risk for strokes, particularly in childhood. Studies indicate that **10% of children with sickle cell disease** will experience a stroke by the age of 20. The risk of stroke is higher among those with sickle cell disease who have had multiple pain crises or who have a history of transient ischemic attacks (TIAs).

Types of Strokes in Sickle Cell Disease

There are two primary types of strokes that occur in individuals with sickle cell disease:

1. **Ischemic Stroke**: This type occurs when the blood flow to the brain is blocked due to a clot formed by sickle-shaped cells obstructing a blood vessel. Ischemic strokes can result in neurological deficits, including difficulty speaking, paralysis, and loss of motor skills.
2. **Hemorrhagic Stroke**: This type of stroke occurs when a blood vessel in the brain bursts, often as a result of weakened blood vessels caused by sickle cell disease. Hemorrhagic strokes can lead to severe damage to the brain, including loss of function and even death.

Preventing and Managing Stroke in Sickle Cell Disease

Preventing strokes is one of the most critical aspects of managing sickle cell disease, particularly in children. Regular screening for stroke risk factors—such as transcranial Doppler ultrasound (TCD)—is standard practice in many healthcare centers for children with sickle cell disease. This test measures blood flow in the brain's arteries and can identify children at high risk for stroke.

For those at high risk, doctors may recommend **blood transfusions** to reduce the number of sickled red blood cells and improve overall circulation. Some children with sickle cell disease receive regular blood transfusions to reduce stroke risk, particularly if their TCD results indicate they are at high risk.

In cases where a stroke occurs, immediate medical intervention is necessary. Treatments may include surgery to remove the clot or medications to dissolve it, as well as rehabilitation to regain lost function. In some cases, children who have had strokes may need long-term physical therapy, occupational therapy, or speech therapy to recover their motor skills and communication abilities.

Organ Damage: The Silent Consequences of Sickle Cell Disease

In addition to pain crises and strokes, sickle cell disease can cause significant damage to several vital organs due to the ongoing blockage of blood flow. Over time, this reduced oxygen delivery to organs can lead to chronic organ dysfunction and failure. Commonly affected organs include the **spleen**, **liver**, **kidneys**, **lungs**, and **heart**.

Spleen Damage (Splenic Sequestration)

The spleen plays a crucial role in filtering bacteria from the blood and storing red blood cells. In sickle cell disease, repeated episodes of blood flow blockage can cause the spleen to become enlarged (splenomegaly) and eventually become nonfunctional, a condition known as **autosplenectomy**. This leads to an increased risk of infection, especially in young children, making vaccination and prophylactic antibiotics essential.

Kidney Damage (Renal Failure)

Sickle cell disease can lead to kidney damage through various mechanisms, including impaired blood flow, chronic inflammation, and the buildup of waste products. The kidneys are responsible for filtering the blood and maintaining fluid balance, and when they become damaged, individuals may experience **kidney failure**. This can necessitate dialysis or even a kidney transplant in severe cases.

Lung Complications (Acute Chest Syndrome)

Another severe complication of sickle cell disease is **acute chest syndrome (ACS)**, a life-threatening condition that involves chest pain, difficulty breathing, fever, and abnormal lung function. ACS is often triggered by infection, fat embolism, or blood clots and can lead to long-term lung damage if left untreated. Individuals with SCD are also at higher risk for **pulmonary hypertension**, which can exacerbate heart and lung problems.

Heart Problems (Cardiomyopathy)

The heart, working under constant strain from the circulatory issues caused by sickle cell disease, may eventually become damaged. Chronic anemia, persistent pain, and lung complications can all contribute to the development of **cardiomyopathy** (a condition in which the heart muscle weakens and loses its ability to pump blood efficiently). Over time, this can lead to **heart failure**, requiring medical interventions such as medications, lifestyle changes, and sometimes heart transplants.

Managing Health: The Road to Better Quality of Life

Living with sickle cell disease is undoubtedly challenging, but with modern medical interventions, patients can manage symptoms and improve their quality of life. Key components of managing SCD include:

- **Regular Check-ups**: People with sickle cell disease require routine monitoring to assess organ function, detect early complications, and adjust treatment plans.
- **Pain Management**: Learning to cope with chronic pain is essential for individuals with SCD. Support from healthcare providers, family, and peers can help individuals manage both physical and emotional pain.
- **Preventative Care**: Vaccination against pneumonia, meningitis, and other infections is critical for people with sickle cell disease, as they are more susceptible to infections due to spleen damage.
- **Hydration and Lifestyle**: Maintaining hydration, avoiding extreme temperatures, and managing stress can help reduce the frequency of pain crises and improve overall health.
- **Psychosocial Support**: Living with a chronic illness can take a toll on mental health, so psychological support, whether through counseling or peer support groups, is important for individuals and their families.

Conclusion

Sickle cell disease is a multifaceted disorder that affects individuals in profound ways. The pain crises, strokes, and organ damage that often accompany SCD present ongoing challenges for patients and healthcare providers alike. However, with advancements in treatment, early detection, and ongoing research, there is hope for better management and, in some cases, a cure. The resilience and determination of those living with sickle cell disease continue to inspire communities around the world to fight for better care, better treatments, and a brighter future.

Chapter 19

Blood Transfusions and Bone Marrow Transplants: Life-Saving Treatments for Sickle Cell Disease

Sickle cell disease (SCD) remains one of the most challenging genetic disorders to manage, given the wide range of complications and symptoms it causes. Despite advances in medical treatment, individuals with SCD often endure frequent painful crises, organ damage, and an increased risk of life-threatening complications like stroke and infection. However, there are life-saving treatments available that can improve the quality of life and even offer a potential cure for some patients. Among the most important of these treatments are blood transfusions and bone marrow transplants, which have been proven to significantly reduce the frequency and severity of complications in many individuals with sickle cell disease.

In this chapter, we will explore the roles that **blood transfusions** and **bone marrow transplants** play in managing sickle cell disease, detailing how these therapies work, their benefits, potential risks, and the current state of research in the field.

Blood Transfusions: A Lifeline for Many Sickle Cell Patients

Blood transfusions are one of the most common and effective treatments for sickle cell disease, particularly for those experiencing frequent and severe complications. The goal of a transfusion is to increase the number of healthy red blood cells in circulation, thereby diluting the sickled cells and improving overall oxygen delivery to tissues. Blood transfusions can help manage a range of SCD-related issues, including anemia, stroke prevention, and the reduction of pain crises.

How Blood Transfusions Work in Sickle Cell Disease

In a typical blood transfusion for sickle cell disease, a patient receives red blood cells from a donor, which are then introduced into the bloodstream. The healthy donor cells replace a portion of the sickled red blood cells, leading to improved blood flow and oxygen delivery to the body. Transfusions can be either **simple** or **exchange** transfusions:

- **Simple Transfusion**: In a simple transfusion, the patient receives blood from a donor, which increases the overall number of red blood cells in the bloodstream. The sickled cells are not specifically removed, but the transfusion helps dilute them.
- **Exchange Transfusion**: This procedure is more specialized. It involves removing a portion of the patient's blood and replacing it with healthy donor blood. Exchange transfusions are often used to treat more severe complications such as stroke prevention or to prepare a patient for surgery. The goal of exchange transfusion is to reduce the percentage of sickle cells in the blood and replace them with normal red blood cells, which significantly improves circulation.

Benefits of Blood Transfusions for Sickle Cell Disease

The benefits of blood transfusions for sickle cell patients are vast. Key advantages include:

- **Reduced Pain Crises**: Transfusions reduce the number of sickled red blood cells in circulation, which can decrease the frequency and intensity of painful vaso-occlusive crises.
- **Prevention of Stroke**: Blood transfusions can reduce the risk of stroke in children with sickle cell disease. By increasing the number of healthy red blood cells and improving blood flow to the brain, transfusions help prevent the blockages that can lead to stroke.
- **Treatment of Anemia**: Many individuals with sickle cell disease suffer from chronic anemia due to the destruction of sickle-shaped red blood cells. Blood transfusions help restore healthy red blood cell levels, improving symptoms such as fatigue and weakness.
- **Management of Organ Damage**: Regular transfusions can help reduce organ damage caused by poor blood circulation. By increasing the number of normal red blood cells, transfusions help prevent further damage to the kidneys, liver, spleen, and other vital organs.
- **Support During Acute Crises**: In the event of an acute complication, such as acute chest syndrome or splenic sequestration, blood transfusions can help stabilize the patient and provide essential support to the body during the crisis.

Risks and Challenges of Blood Transfusions

Despite their benefits, blood transfusions come with potential risks, especially when they are performed frequently. Some of the main risks associated with blood transfusions include:

- **Iron Overload**: One of the most common side effects of frequent blood transfusions is **iron overload**. The body cannot easily excrete the excess iron in transfused blood, and over time, this can accumulate in vital organs such as the liver, heart, and endocrine glands. To prevent iron overload, patients typically undergo **chelation therapy**, a treatment designed to remove excess iron from the body.
- **Alloimmunization**: Alloimmunization occurs when a patient's immune system recognizes foreign red blood cells (from the donor blood) and develops antibodies against them. This can make it harder for the patient to receive compatible blood in the future, which can complicate the treatment process.
- **Infections**: Although rigorous screening processes are in place to ensure that donor blood is free from infectious agents, there is still a small risk of transmitting infections through blood transfusions. This risk has significantly decreased over the years due to improvements in screening and blood safety measures.
- **Volume Overload**: In some cases, receiving multiple transfusions can lead to **volume overload**, where the circulatory system becomes overwhelmed with the additional blood volume, potentially leading to complications such as heart failure.

While blood transfusions are a cornerstone of SCD treatment, they are not a permanent solution. Many patients require long-term transfusions, which can have cumulative effects on their health over time.

Bone Marrow Transplants: A Potential Cure for Sickle Cell Disease

Bone marrow transplants (BMT), also known as **hematopoietic stem cell transplants,** offer the potential for a curative treatment for sickle cell disease. This procedure involves replacing a patient's bone marrow (which produces the defective red blood cells) with healthy stem cells from a matched donor, typically a sibling or unrelated donor. The new stem cells begin to produce normal red blood cells, potentially curing the patient of sickle cell disease.

How Bone Marrow Transplants Work

Bone marrow transplants involve several steps, beginning with the **conditioning regimen**, which may include chemotherapy or radiation. This step is necessary to destroy the patient's defective bone marrow and suppress the immune system to prevent rejection of the transplanted cells. Once the conditioning is complete, the patient receives an infusion of healthy stem cells from a compatible donor.

The transplanted stem cells migrate to the patient's bone marrow and begin producing new blood cells, including red blood cells with normal hemoglobin. Over time, this process gradually replaces the sickle-shaped cells with healthy red blood cells, offering a potential cure for sickle cell disease.

Benefits of Bone Marrow Transplant for Sickle Cell Disease

A bone marrow transplant offers the possibility of a cure for sickle cell disease, which is a life-changing event for many patients. Some key benefits include:

- **Permanent Cure**: In some cases, a bone marrow transplant can completely cure sickle cell disease, eliminating the need for ongoing treatments such as blood transfusions and pain management.
- **Improved Quality of Life**: Following a successful transplant, patients can experience a significant improvement in their quality of life, with a reduced risk of pain crises, stroke, and organ damage.
- **Potential for Lifelong Health**: Once the transplant has been successful, patients can potentially live a life free of the debilitating effects of sickle cell disease.

Risks and Challenges of Bone Marrow Transplants

Despite the potential benefits, bone marrow transplants come with significant risks, especially in patients who are older or have other health complications. These risks include:

- **Graft-Versus-Host Disease (GVHD)**: One of the most serious risks of bone marrow transplant is graft-versus-host disease, which occurs when the transplanted donor cells attack the patient's tissues. GVHD can range from mild to life-threatening and can affect the skin, liver, gastrointestinal system, and other organs.

- **Rejection of the Transplanted Cells**: In some cases, the patient's immune system may reject the transplanted stem cells, causing the procedure to fail.
- **Infection Risk**: After a transplant, patients undergo immunosuppressive treatment to prevent rejection of the transplanted cells, which leaves them vulnerable to infections. Careful monitoring and infection control measures are essential to minimize this risk.
- **Difficulty Finding a Match**: The success of a bone marrow transplant depends heavily on finding a suitable donor. For many patients, especially those from minority ethnic groups, finding a compatible match can be a significant challenge, and not all patients are eligible for this treatment.
- **Cost and Accessibility**: Bone marrow transplants are complex procedures that require significant financial resources and access to specialized healthcare facilities. For many families, the cost of the procedure, along with the required post-transplant care, can be prohibitively expensive.

Current Research and Future Directions

Research into bone marrow transplants for sickle cell disease is ongoing. New techniques, such as **gene therapy** and **gene editing**, are being explored as potential ways to improve the success rate of bone marrow transplants and make the procedure more accessible to a wider population. Gene therapy involves modifying the patient's own cells to produce healthy hemoglobin, offering an alternative to traditional bone marrow transplants. Clinical trials are currently underway to evaluate the safety and efficacy of these groundbreaking approaches.

Conclusion

Blood transfusions and bone marrow transplants are powerful tools in the management of sickle cell disease, offering relief from complications and, in some cases, the possibility of a cure. While blood transfusions provide critical short-term benefits by improving circulation and reducing pain crises, bone marrow transplants offer the hope of long-term remission or even complete cure. Both treatments come with their own risks and challenges, but with ongoing research and advancements in medical technology, the future for individuals with sickle cell disease looks brighter than ever. Through the continued pursuit of better treatments and potential cures, there is hope that one day, sickle cell disease may be eradicated altogether, providing future generations with a life free from its burdens.

Chapter 20

Thalassemia: The Hemoglobin Deficiency

Thalassemia is a group of inherited blood disorders that affect the body's ability to produce hemoglobin properly, leading to anemia and a range of associated complications. Unlike other forms of anemia, which may be caused by nutritional deficiencies or external factors, thalassemia is genetic, passed down from parents to their children. This condition involves the underproduction or abnormal production of hemoglobin, a crucial protein in red blood cells responsible for transporting oxygen throughout the body. As a result, individuals with thalassemia often face a variety of health challenges, including fatigue, weakness, and, in severe cases, organ damage due to iron overload.

In this chapter, we will delve into the complexities of thalassemia, exploring its types, causes, symptoms, diagnostic methods, and treatment options. We will also discuss the genetic inheritance patterns of thalassemia and how advances in medical research and treatment are improving the quality of life for those affected by this disorder.

What is Thalassemia?

Thalassemia is a blood disorder caused by mutations in the genes responsible for producing hemoglobin, the protein in red blood cells that binds oxygen and transports it throughout the body. Hemoglobin consists of four protein chains: two alpha chains and two beta chains. Thalassemia occurs when there is an issue with the production of either the alpha or beta chains, which leads to the production of defective hemoglobin.

There are two main types of thalassemia, based on which part of the hemoglobin molecule is affected:

1. **Alpha Thalassemia**: In alpha thalassemia, the body is unable to produce enough alpha globin chains, which are essential for the formation of hemoglobin. There are two genes that control the production of alpha globin chains, and individuals with alpha thalassemia inherit mutations in one or more of these genes. The severity of the disorder depends on how many of these genes are affected.

2. **Beta Thalassemia**: In beta thalassemia, there is a deficiency or complete absence of beta globin chains. The beta globin genes are responsible for producing the beta globin chains that pair with the alpha chains to form hemoglobin. This type of thalassemia can be classified into three major forms based on severity:
     - **Beta Thalassemia Minor**: This is a mild form of the disease that often causes no or very mild symptoms. It occurs when one beta globin gene is mutated while the other remains normal.
     - **Beta Thalassemia Intermedia**: This form is more severe than beta thalassemia minor but not as severe as thalassemia major. Patients may require occasional blood transfusions.
     - **Beta Thalassemia Major (Cooley's Anemia)**: This is the most severe form of the disease and requires regular blood transfusions from a young age. Patients with this form often experience significant complications, including growth delays, bone deformities, and organ damage due to iron overload.

Genetic Inheritance of Thalassemia

Thalassemia is inherited in an **autosomal recessive** manner, meaning that both parents must carry the gene mutation for a child to inherit the disorder. If a person inherits only one mutated gene, they are considered a **carrier**, and they typically do not show symptoms, but they can pass the gene on to their offspring. Carriers of thalassemia may not even realize they have the condition unless they undergo genetic testing.

- **If both parents are carriers (heterozygous)**, each of their children has a:
     - 25% chance of inheriting two normal genes and being unaffected.
     - 50% chance of inheriting one mutated gene and being a carrier.
     - 25% chance of inheriting two mutated genes, resulting in thalassemia.

If one parent has thalassemia major and the other is a carrier or unaffected, their children have a higher risk of inheriting the condition.

Symptoms and Complications of Thalassemia

The severity of thalassemia symptoms depends on the type of thalassemia an individual has and whether they inherit one or two copies of the mutated gene. Symptoms generally result from the inadequate production of hemoglobin and the resulting inability of red blood cells to carry oxygen efficiently.

Common symptoms of thalassemia include:

- **Fatigue and Weakness**: The reduced number of red blood cells and ineffective hemoglobin production lead to insufficient oxygen transport throughout the body, causing tiredness and general weakness.
- **Paleness (Pallor)**: Due to anemia, individuals with thalassemia often appear paler than normal, particularly in the skin and the inside of the eyes.
- **Enlarged Spleen and Liver (Splenomegaly and Hepatomegaly)**: The body's attempt to compensate for the lack of effective red blood cells leads to overproduction in the bone marrow, which can cause the spleen and liver to enlarge.
- **Bone Deformities**: Severe thalassemia (beta thalassemia major) can cause bone marrow expansion, leading to abnormal bone growth and deformities, particularly in the face and skull.
- **Delayed Growth and Development**: Children with severe forms of thalassemia may experience delayed physical and sexual growth due to chronic anemia.
- **Heart Problems**: Chronic anemia and iron overload can eventually affect the heart, leading to complications such as heart failure and arrhythmias.

In some cases, thalassemia can lead to severe complications, including **organ failure, growth retardation, gallstones**, and **bone fractures. Iron overload** is another serious issue in thalassemia, especially in patients who undergo regular blood transfusions. Excess iron can accumulate in vital organs such as the liver, heart, and endocrine glands, leading to damage if not properly managed.

Diagnosing Thalassemia

Thalassemia is typically diagnosed through a combination of blood tests, genetic testing, and family history. Some of the key diagnostic tools include:

- **Complete Blood Count (CBC)**: This is usually the first test done to check for anemia. In thalassemia, the CBC may show a reduced red blood cell count and small (microcytic), pale (hypochromic) red blood cells.
- **Hemoglobin Electrophoresis**: This test helps identify abnormal forms of hemoglobin in the blood. It is a crucial diagnostic tool for confirming thalassemia, as it can detect changes in hemoglobin composition that indicate thalassemia or other hemoglobinopathies.

- **Genetic Testing**: To confirm the presence of specific mutations in the alpha or beta globin genes, genetic testing is often used. This is especially important for carrier testing or prenatal diagnosis.
- **Iron Studies**: In patients with thalassemia who undergo regular transfusions, iron levels may be monitored to detect iron overload, which can be managed with chelation therapy.

Treatment of Thalassemia

There is no universal cure for thalassemia, but various treatments can help manage symptoms and improve quality of life. The treatment plan depends on the severity of the disease and the individual's specific health needs.

1. Blood Transfusions

For individuals with severe thalassemia (especially beta thalassemia major), regular blood transfusions are essential. Transfusions increase the number of normal red blood cells in circulation, alleviating symptoms of anemia and improving oxygen delivery to tissues. However, long-term transfusions can lead to **iron overload**, which must be managed with other treatments.

2. Iron Chelation Therapy

Since blood transfusions can lead to iron buildup in the body, **iron chelation therapy** is used to remove excess iron and prevent organ damage. Chelating agents, such as **deferoxamine, deferasirox,** or **deferiprone**, bind to the excess iron in the body and help excrete it through urine or stool.

3. Bone Marrow and Stem Cell Transplants

For some patients, a **bone marrow transplant** (also called **hematopoietic stem cell transplant**) offers a potential cure for thalassemia. This procedure involves replacing the patient's defective bone marrow with healthy stem cells from a matched donor, which can produce normal red blood cells. Bone marrow transplants are typically recommended for patients with severe forms of the disease and who have a suitable donor.

4. Gene Therapy

Gene therapy is a cutting-edge treatment that aims to cure thalassemia by introducing a healthy version of the mutated gene into a patient's cells. Research in gene therapy for thalassemia is still ongoing, but early results have shown promise in providing a long-term solution for some patients. This approach has the potential to reduce or eliminate the need for regular blood transfusions.

5. Supportive Care

Individuals with thalassemia may also benefit from **supportive care** to manage symptoms and complications. This may include pain management, physical therapy, growth hormone treatment for children, and other interventions to improve overall health.

Living with Thalassemia

While thalassemia is a chronic condition, with proper medical management, many individuals with the disorder can lead relatively normal lives. However, the need for ongoing care and frequent medical appointments can be burdensome, and the emotional toll of the disease should not be underestimated. Psychological support, counseling, and support groups are important components of comprehensive care for people with thalassemia.

Conclusion

Thalassemia is a complex genetic blood disorder that can significantly impact the health and well-being of affected individuals. While there is currently no permanent cure for the disorder, advances in treatment options, including blood transfusions, iron chelation, stem cell transplants, and potential gene therapy, are improving the outlook for those with thalassemia.

By understanding the condition, its symptoms, and the available treatments, people with thalassemia can better manage their health and reduce the impact of this lifelong disease. The continued advancement in medical research holds hope for a brighter future, with the potential for even more effective treatments or a cure for thalassemia on the horizon.

Chapter 21

Living with Thalassemia: Challenges and Advances

Living with thalassemia presents a unique set of challenges for individuals and their families, as the disorder is lifelong and requires ongoing care. The constant management of blood levels, the regular need for medical appointments, and the emotional and physical toll of the disease can weigh heavily on those affected. Yet, despite these difficulties, many people with thalassemia lead fulfilling lives, thanks to advances in treatment and a growing understanding of the disorder. This chapter explores what it's like to live with thalassemia, the hurdles individuals face on a daily basis, and the promising advances in gene therapy that offer hope for the future.

The Daily Struggles of Living with Thalassemia

Thalassemia impacts various aspects of daily life, depending on the severity of the condition. For individuals with the most severe forms of thalassemia, such as beta thalassemia major, living with the disease often means adhering to a strict regimen of medical treatments. These can include frequent blood transfusions, iron chelation therapy, and constant monitoring of iron levels. Even for those with milder forms, such as beta thalassemia minor, the condition can still affect daily life, though the impact is typically less severe.

Regular Blood Transfusions

For people with beta thalassemia major, blood transfusions are often a lifeline. These transfusions are necessary to maintain red blood cell counts at levels sufficient for carrying oxygen throughout the body. However, receiving regular transfusions can lead to iron overload—a serious complication of thalassemia. To counter this, individuals must also undergo **iron chelation therapy**, which involves the use of medications to remove excess iron from the body.

The requirement for frequent blood transfusions can be disruptive, often leading to hospital visits every few weeks. For children with thalassemia, this schedule can be particularly challenging, requiring them to miss school and participate in treatments that are often uncomfortable. For adults, the strain of regular medical appointments can affect work, social life, and family responsibilities.

Iron Chelation Therapy

Iron chelation therapy is a critical aspect of thalassemia management, particularly for individuals who undergo regular blood transfusions. This therapy helps prevent the dangerous buildup of iron in the body, which can damage vital organs such as the heart, liver, and pancreas.

While chelation therapy has significantly improved the life expectancy and quality of life for people with thalassemia, it is not without its challenges. Chelating agents, such as **deferoxamine, deferasirox**, and **deferiprone**, can cause side effects such as nausea, gastrointestinal distress, and even organ toxicity if not properly monitored. Some individuals also find it difficult to adhere to the long-term treatment regimens, especially in the case of deferoxamine, which is administered through a subcutaneous pump over several hours, typically every day.

Despite these difficulties, the benefits of iron chelation therapy are immense, as it prevents the fatal consequences of iron buildup, including liver cirrhosis, heart failure, and diabetes.

Emotional and Psychological Impact

The emotional burden of living with a chronic, lifelong illness like thalassemia is significant. The constant need for medical interventions, the uncertainty of health complications, and the awareness of the hereditary nature of the disease can lead to feelings of anxiety, stress, and isolation.

For parents of children with thalassemia, the fear of passing the genetic condition on to future generations adds another layer of complexity. The burden of ensuring that their children follow strict medical regimens, while also providing them with a sense of normalcy, can create emotional strain. Similarly, adults with thalassemia may experience frustration and sadness, particularly if they are unable to live the same life as their peers due to the limitations of the disease.

Psychological support, counseling, and community networks are critical for individuals living with thalassemia, helping them navigate the emotional toll of the condition. Support groups, both in-person and online, provide a safe space for individuals to share experiences, advice, and encouragement.

Treatment Strategies and Their Impact

While there is no cure for thalassemia at present, significant strides have been made in treatment options, particularly in terms of **blood transfusions**, **iron chelation**, and **bone marrow transplantation**.

Blood Transfusions and Bone Marrow Transplants

Blood transfusions remain the cornerstone of treatment for severe thalassemia. These transfusions help to alleviate the symptoms of anemia by boosting red blood cell counts, which in turn improves oxygen delivery to tissues and reduces fatigue.

For those with severe forms of the disease who cannot manage with transfusions alone, a **bone marrow or stem cell transplant** offers the potential for a cure. This treatment involves replacing the patient's faulty bone marrow with healthy stem cells from a matched donor, allowing the body to produce healthy red blood cells on its own. Although this procedure offers the hope of a normal life, it is not without risks. Bone marrow transplants require the use of **immunosuppressive drugs** to prevent rejection, and the procedure can result in complications such as infections, graft-versus-host disease, and long-term organ damage.

For many, bone marrow transplants are a last-resort treatment option, especially as the availability of matched donors is often limited. However, for those fortunate enough to undergo a successful transplant, it can significantly change the course of their disease.

Advances in Gene Therapy: A Ray of Hope

In recent years, **gene therapy** has emerged as one of the most promising treatment options for thalassemia. The goal of gene therapy is to correct the underlying genetic mutations that cause the disease. By introducing a normal copy of the mutated gene responsible for hemoglobin production into the patient's cells, researchers hope to enable the body to produce normal hemoglobin without the need for frequent blood transfusions or iron chelation.

Several clinical trials are underway to test gene therapy for thalassemia, with encouraging results. Some individuals who have undergone gene therapy have shown substantial improvement, with their bodies producing normal hemoglobin levels and reducing their dependence on blood transfusions. However, gene therapy is still in its experimental stages and is not yet widely available as a standard treatment.

The potential for gene therapy to revolutionize thalassemia treatment is immense. If successful on a broader scale, gene therapy could eliminate the need for lifelong blood transfusions, iron chelation, and bone marrow transplants. It would offer a more permanent solution to thalassemia, potentially curing the disease and allowing patients to live free from the burdens of ongoing medical treatment.

Living Well with Thalassemia: The Importance of Holistic Care

While the physical management of thalassemia is critical, living well with the disorder also requires a focus on holistic care. This includes regular monitoring of blood levels, emotional support, and maintaining a healthy lifestyle. People with thalassemia are encouraged to follow a balanced diet rich in nutrients to support their overall health and prevent complications. Maintaining regular exercise routines, when possible, can help manage fatigue and improve cardiovascular health, which is particularly important in light of the potential heart problems that can arise from the disease.

Psychosocial support is just as crucial as medical treatment. Living with thalassemia means navigating both the medical and emotional challenges of the condition. Support groups, counseling, and mental health care can help individuals and families cope with the stress of living with a chronic illness.

Conclusion: A Brighter Future Ahead

Living with thalassemia is undoubtedly challenging, but advancements in medical treatments, such as blood transfusions, iron chelation therapy, and stem cell transplants, have vastly improved the prognosis for many individuals. The emergence of gene therapy offers hope for a future where thalassemia may no longer be a lifelong burden.

As research continues, and more individuals gain access to cutting-edge treatments, those living with thalassemia may one day experience a world in which the disease is no longer a limiting factor. For now, the ongoing support of healthcare providers, families, and the global thalassemia community remains a vital part of managing this condition, helping people to live full, active lives despite the challenges they face. Through perseverance, advancements, and the shared strength of the thalassemia community, there is hope for a future without the daily struggles of this blood disorder.

Chapter 22

Understanding Deep Vein Thrombosis (DVT)

Blood clotting is a natural process that helps our body stop bleeding when we are injured. However, when clotting occurs at the wrong time or in the wrong place, it can lead to serious health complications. One such condition is **Deep Vein Thrombosis** (DVT), a condition where a blood clot forms in one of the deep veins of the body, usually in the legs. This chapter delves into what DVT is, how it forms, its causes, risk factors, symptoms, potential complications, and the relationship between DVT and other health conditions like heart disease, obesity, and more.

What is Deep Vein Thrombosis (DVT)?

Deep vein thrombosis is the formation of a blood clot, also known as a **thrombus**, in one of the deep veins of the body. The most common site for DVT is in the lower legs, though it can also occur in other parts of the body, including the thighs, pelvis, or arms. These deep veins are located beneath the surface of the skin and carry blood back to the heart.

A thrombus that forms in a deep vein can vary in size, from a small clot that causes no symptoms to a larger one that can cause significant pain, swelling, and even more serious complications. In some cases, the clot may remain in place and not cause major issues, but in many situations, the clot can break loose and travel to other parts of the body, such as the lungs, where it can cause a potentially life-threatening condition known as a **pulmonary embolism (PE).**

DVT often develops without clear symptoms, making it difficult to diagnose without proper testing. If left untreated, however, it can lead to long-term health problems, including **post-thrombotic syndrome**, which is a condition characterized by chronic pain, swelling, and discomfort in the affected leg.

How DVT Forms: The Physiology Behind Blood Clots

The process of blood clotting is essential for healing when we suffer injuries. The body uses a complex system of proteins, platelets, and other factors to form clots, which prevent excessive bleeding. However, when this clotting process is triggered inappropriately, it can cause problems like DVT.

Blood clots typically form in the veins when three factors come into play, known as **Virchow's Triad**:

1. **Stasis of Blood Flow:** When blood flow becomes slow or stagnant, as can happen when a person is immobile for extended periods (such as during long flights, hospital stays, or bed rest), the likelihood of clot formation increases. This is especially true in the lower limbs, where gravity causes blood to pool and circulate less efficiently.
2. **Hypercoagulability:** This refers to the increased tendency of blood to clot. Certain medical conditions or genetic factors can make a person's blood more prone to clotting. Conditions like **cancer**, **pregnancy**, and **autoimmune disorders**, as well as certain medications (e.g., hormonal contraceptives), can cause hypercoagulability. Additionally, genetic mutations that affect clotting factors can also lead to a higher risk of DVT.
3. **Vessel Injury:** Injury to the walls of blood vessels, such as from surgery, trauma, or inflammation, can initiate clotting. A common cause of vein damage is surgery, particularly surgeries of the hips, knees, or legs, which increase the risk of DVT due to both immobilization and the surgical trauma to blood vessels.

Together, these three factors—stasis of blood flow, hypercoagulability, and vessel injury—create the perfect conditions for a clot to form and remain in the deep veins of the body, potentially leading to DVT.

Risk Factors for DVT

Several factors increase the likelihood of developing DVT. These risk factors can be broadly categorized into lifestyle-related factors, medical conditions, and genetic predispositions:

1. Prolonged Immobility

Long periods of immobility are among the most common risk factors for DVT. Extended sitting, such as on long-haul flights, car trips, or in a sedentary job, can slow blood flow in the veins of the legs, allowing clots to form. Hospitalization for surgery or illness, particularly if the individual is confined to bed rest for an extended period, also increases the risk of developing DVT.

2. Obesity

Obesity is another significant risk factor for DVT. Excess body weight puts additional pressure on the veins in the lower body, impairing circulation. Furthermore, people with obesity often have other associated conditions such as **diabetes, hypertension**, and **heart disease**, which compound the risk. The presence of fatty tissue can also hinder the movement of blood, making it more likely for clotting to occur.

3. Age

As people age, the risk of developing DVT increases. Older adults have more rigid, less flexible veins, which may impede blood flow. In addition, older adults are more likely to suffer from conditions like heart disease, varicose veins, or mobility issues that contribute to clot formation.

4. Pregnancy

Pregnant women are at a higher risk for DVT due to hormonal changes that increase blood clotting, as well as the physical changes that occur during pregnancy, including increased pressure on the veins from the growing uterus. The risk remains elevated for up to six weeks postpartum, particularly if the woman has had a cesarean section or other complications during childbirth.

5. Medical Conditions

Certain medical conditions can increase the risk of DVT, including **heart disease, stroke, cancer, inflammatory bowel disease (IBD)**, and **kidney disease**. Cancer, in particular, is strongly associated with a higher risk of DVT, especially in those undergoing chemotherapy or other treatments that may increase clotting tendencies.

6. Genetic Predispositions

Some people are born with genetic mutations that affect their blood's clotting ability. Known as **inherited thrombophilia**, these conditions increase the risk of abnormal clot formation. Some common inherited blood disorders that predispose individuals to DVT include **Factor V Leiden mutation, prothrombin gene mutation**, and **protein C or protein S deficiency**.

Symptoms of DVT

DVT is sometimes referred to as the "silent killer" because many people do not exhibit any symptoms. However, when symptoms do occur, they are typically localized to the affected leg and may include:

- **Swelling**: The affected leg may become noticeably swollen, particularly around the calf area.
- **Pain or Tenderness**: Pain, aching, or cramping often occurs in the affected leg, especially when standing or walking.
- **Red or Discolored Skin**: The skin over the clot may become red, warm, or have a bluish tint.
- **Increased Leg Temperature**: The affected leg may feel warmer than usual.

In severe cases, DVT may be associated with a **pulmonary embolism (PE)**, a life-threatening complication that occurs when a blood clot breaks free and travels to the lungs, blocking blood flow. Symptoms of a PE include sudden shortness of breath, chest pain, rapid heart rate, and coughing up blood.

Complications of DVT

The most serious complication of DVT is **pulmonary embolism (PE)**. A blood clot that breaks free from the vein and travels to the lungs can block one of the pulmonary arteries, leading to impaired blood flow and oxygenation in the lungs. This is a medical emergency and requires immediate attention. Symptoms of a PE include severe chest pain, difficulty breathing, and coughing up blood. Without treatment, a pulmonary embolism can be fatal.

Another long-term complication of DVT is **post-thrombotic syndrome (PTS)**, which occurs in approximately 20-50% of people who have experienced a DVT. PTS involves chronic pain, swelling, and skin changes in the affected leg, which can significantly impact a person's quality of life. The damage to the veins caused by the clot can impair normal circulation, leading to these persistent symptoms.

Diagnosis and Treatment of DVT

The diagnosis of DVT usually involves a combination of physical examination, medical history review, and diagnostic tests. A common test for DVT is **ultrasound**, which uses sound waves to create an image of the blood flow in the veins and detect the presence of a clot. In some cases, a **D-dimer test**, which measures the levels of a substance released when a blood clot breaks up, may also be used to assess the likelihood of a clot.

Once diagnosed, DVT is typically treated with blood-thinning medications, also known as **anticoagulants**, which help prevent the clot from growing and reduce the risk of it traveling to the lungs. **Compression stockings** may also be recommended to reduce swelling and improve blood circulation. In severe cases, procedures such as **thrombolysis** (using medication to dissolve the clot) or **surgical removal of the clot** may be necessary.

Prevention of DVT

Prevention of DVT involves reducing risk factors and promoting healthy circulation. This can include:

- Staying active and avoiding prolonged immobility.
- Using **compression stockings** to improve blood flow during long periods of sitting.
- Taking regular breaks to stand and walk if you have a sedentary job.
- For individuals at higher risk, taking prescribed **anticoagulant medications** and following your doctor's advice.

Conclusion

Deep vein thrombosis is a serious condition that can lead to severe complications if not properly managed. It often occurs silently, without noticeable symptoms, and can cause life-threatening consequences if left untreated. Understanding the risk factors, symptoms, and treatment options is essential for preventing and managing DVT. With prompt diagnosis and appropriate treatment, many people with DVT can lead healthy, active lives, avoiding the complications of pulmonary embolism and post-thrombotic syndrome. As with many health conditions, awareness, early detection, and prevention are the key to reducing the risk of severe outcomes.

Chapter 23

Pulmonary Embolism: The Silent Killer

A pulmonary embolism (PE) is one of the most severe and life-threatening complications of deep vein thrombosis (DVT). When a blood clot that forms in a deep vein — most commonly in the legs — breaks loose and travels through the bloodstream, it can lodge in the lungs, obstructing blood flow and causing significant damage. Known as the **silent killer**, pulmonary embolism often strikes without warning, making it a medical emergency that requires immediate intervention. In this chapter, we will explore the pathophysiology of pulmonary embolism, its symptoms, the risks associated with untreated DVT, the diagnosis process, treatment options, and the critical importance of early detection.

What is Pulmonary Embolism?

A pulmonary embolism occurs when a blood clot, often originating from the deep veins of the legs or pelvis (known as **DVT**), breaks free and travels through the bloodstream to the lungs. The clot — now referred to as an **embolus** — can block one of the pulmonary arteries or its branches, restricting blood flow to the lung tissue and leading to oxygen deprivation in the affected area. This blockage causes the lung tissue to suffer from lack of oxygen, potentially leading to **cardiovascular collapse** or **death** if not treated promptly.

The size and location of the clot will determine the severity of the pulmonary embolism. A **small clot** might cause minor symptoms and be absorbed by the body with minimal harm, while a **large clot** can obstruct a major pulmonary artery, resulting in severe respiratory distress, shock, and even death.

How Pulmonary Embolism Develops

Pulmonary embolism is typically a secondary condition, resulting from an untreated or undiagnosed DVT. When a blood clot forms in the veins of the legs, it is usually due to factors such as prolonged immobility, blood clotting disorders, or trauma. If a clot is not identified or treated, it may grow larger over time, causing increased risk. Eventually, the clot may dislodge and enter the bloodstream, traveling to the heart, and then into the lungs.

Once in the lungs, the clot can obstruct the pulmonary arteries, limiting the lung's ability to transfer oxygen into the bloodstream. This process severely disrupts normal circulation and causes complications, some of which can be fatal if the blockage is not cleared in time.

Symptoms of Pulmonary Embolism

The symptoms of pulmonary embolism can vary greatly depending on the size of the clot, the location of the blockage, and the individual's overall health. In some cases, PE can develop suddenly and dramatically, while in others, it may evolve more gradually. Recognizing the symptoms early is critical for improving outcomes, as prompt medical intervention can significantly reduce the risk of fatal complications.

Common Symptoms of Pulmonary Embolism Include:

- **Sudden Shortness of Breath**: One of the hallmark signs of PE is sudden, unexplained difficulty breathing. This can range from mild to severe, depending on the extent of the blockage.
- **Chest Pain**: Often described as sharp or stabbing, chest pain associated with pulmonary embolism may worsen with deep breathing or coughing. In some cases, the pain may resemble that of a heart attack, making the condition difficult to diagnose without medical tests.
- **Coughing (with or without Blood)**: A persistent cough that may produce **blood-streaked sputum** or even lead to coughing up blood is another potential sign of pulmonary embolism.
- **Rapid Heart Rate (Tachycardia)**: In response to the reduced oxygen levels in the bloodstream, the heart may begin to beat faster than usual to compensate for the impaired blood flow.
- **Dizziness or Lightheadedness**: A PE can cause a sudden drop in blood pressure, leading to dizziness, fainting, or near-fainting episodes.
- **Swelling in the Leg**: If the PE is associated with DVT, there may be swelling, warmth, or redness in the affected leg. These symptoms are often an indication that the clot came from a vein in the lower extremity.

It's important to note that the symptoms of pulmonary embolism can be subtle or mimic other conditions, including heart attack, pneumonia, or asthma. For this reason, it is crucial to seek immediate medical attention if these symptoms arise.

Risk Factors and Causes of Pulmonary Embolism

The primary cause of pulmonary embolism is the development of deep vein thrombosis (DVT), but there are several risk factors that make individuals more susceptible to developing PE. Some of these factors include:

1. Prolonged Immobility

Prolonged periods of immobility, such as long-haul flights, extended hospital stays, or bed rest after surgery, can significantly increase the risk of DVT and, consequently, pulmonary embolism. When blood flow slows down, clots can form more easily in the veins of the legs, setting the stage for a potential PE.

2. Pregnancy and Postpartum Period

Pregnant women are more likely to develop blood clots due to hormonal changes that increase blood clotting. Additionally, the pressure from the growing uterus on the veins in the pelvis can slow blood flow and contribute to clot formation. The risk of pulmonary embolism remains elevated for up to six weeks after childbirth.

3. Birth Control Pills or Hormone Replacement Therapy (HRT)

Hormonal medications, such as oral contraceptives or hormone replacement therapy, increase the blood's tendency to clot, which can heighten the risk of developing DVT and, by extension, PE.

4. Surgery

Surgical procedures, particularly those involving the hips, legs, or abdomen, carry an increased risk of blood clots forming in the deep veins. The risks are particularly high when surgery is followed by immobility or prolonged bed rest.

5. Obesity

Excess body weight can contribute to the development of both DVT and PE, as it increases pressure on the veins, leading to poor blood circulation and a higher likelihood of clot formation.

6. Genetic Conditions

Certain inherited conditions, such as **Factor V Leiden** mutation, **antithrombin III deficiency**, or **protein C and S deficiency**, increase the blood's ability to clot, putting individuals at higher risk for both DVT and pulmonary embolism.

7. Cancer

Cancer, particularly cancers of the pancreas, lungs, and gastrointestinal tract, increases the likelihood of clot formation. Additionally, cancer treatments such as chemotherapy can also increase the clotting risk, leading to a greater chance of PE.

Complications of Pulmonary Embolism

Without timely diagnosis and treatment, pulmonary embolism can lead to a range of serious complications, some of which can be fatal. The most dangerous complication is **cardiovascular collapse**, in which the right side of the heart fails due to the increased pressure in the lungs caused by the clot. This can cause a dramatic drop in blood pressure and result in shock, organ failure, and even death.

Other potential complications of pulmonary embolism include:

- **Chronic Pulmonary Hypertension**: Long-term PE can cause high blood pressure in the pulmonary arteries, leading to damage to the heart and lungs.
- **Respiratory Failure**: Severe PE can reduce oxygen levels in the bloodstream to a dangerous degree, leading to respiratory failure.
- **Post-PE Syndrome**: Some people may experience long-term symptoms, including shortness of breath, chest pain, or difficulty exercising, even after the clot has been resolved.

Diagnosis of Pulmonary Embolism

Given the serious nature of pulmonary embolism, quick and accurate diagnosis is essential. Several diagnostic tools are used to confirm the presence of PE, including:

Computed Tomography Pulmonary Angiography (CTPA)

CTPA is the gold standard for diagnosing pulmonary embolism. This imaging test uses a contrast dye to highlight the pulmonary arteries, allowing doctors to detect any blockages in the blood flow.

Ventilation-Perfusion (V/Q) Scan

This imaging test assesses the airflow and blood flow in the lungs to detect any areas where blood flow is obstructed by a clot.

Ultrasound of the Legs

Since DVT is the most common source of pulmonary embolism, doctors may use an ultrasound to detect blood clots in the legs or pelvic veins.

D-dimer Test

The D-dimer test measures the levels of a specific substance released when a clot breaks down. High levels of D-dimer in the blood can indicate the presence of a clot in the body, though further imaging tests are required for a definitive diagnosis.

Treatment of Pulmonary Embolism

Treatment of pulmonary embolism aims to remove or dissolve the clot, restore normal blood flow, and prevent further clot formation. Common treatment options include:

Anticoagulants (Blood Thinners)

The first line of treatment for pulmonary embolism is the administration of blood thinners such as **heparin** or **warfarin**. These medications help prevent existing clots from growing and reduce the risk of new clots forming.

Thrombolytic Therapy

In cases of large or life-threatening pulmonary embolism, thrombolytic medications (clot-busting drugs) may be administered to dissolve the clot more rapidly. This treatment carries a risk of bleeding and is typically used only in severe cases.

Surgical Intervention

In rare cases, when the clot is large and not responsive to medications, surgery may be required to physically remove the clot from the pulmonary artery.

Catheter-directed thrombolysis or **embolectomy** are options that may be considered.

Inferior Vena Cava (IVC) Filter

For individuals who cannot take blood thinners due to other medical conditions, or who have recurrent pulmonary embolisms, an IVC filter may be inserted to prevent clots from traveling to the lungs.

Preventing Pulmonary Embolism

The key to preventing pulmonary embolism is managing the risk factors for DVT and promoting healthy circulation. Some strategies to reduce the risk of PE include:

- **Regular physical activity**: Engaging in regular exercise promotes healthy blood flow and prevents clots from forming.
- **Compression stockings**: These can help prevent blood clots in individuals at high risk for DVT.
- **Medication management**: For individuals at high risk of clotting, anticoagulant medications can help prevent clots from forming.
- **Post-surgery care**: Following surgery, early mobilization and the use of blood thinners can help reduce the risk of DVT and PE.

Conclusion

Pulmonary embolism remains a serious and potentially deadly condition, but with early diagnosis, prompt treatment, and appropriate management, many individuals with PE can recover and return to normal activity. It is crucial for individuals at risk to be aware of the signs and symptoms of pulmonary embolism and to seek immediate medical attention if any warning signs arise. By understanding the risk factors, complications, and available treatment options, individuals can take proactive steps to protect their health and minimize the risk of this silent but deadly disease.

Chapter 24

The Dangers of DVT: Symptoms, Diagnosis, and Prevention

Deep vein thrombosis (DVT) is a potentially life-threatening condition in which a blood clot (thrombus) forms in one of the deep veins of the body, typically in the legs. If left untreated, the clot can travel to the lungs, leading to a pulmonary embolism (PE), a serious complication that can cause death. While DVT may not always present immediate symptoms, it is crucial to understand its early warning signs, diagnostic procedures, and preventive measures in order to reduce the risk of complications.

In this chapter, we will delve into the dangers of DVT, how to recognize its symptoms, and the steps individuals can take to prevent it. Knowledge and vigilance are key to managing the risks associated with DVT and ensuring a healthy circulatory system.

What is Deep Vein Thrombosis (DVT)?

DVT occurs when a blood clot forms in one of the deep veins of the body, most often in the legs. This can happen when the blood flow becomes sluggish, allowing blood to pool and clot. While the condition is more commonly found in the lower extremities, it can also occur in the arms and other parts of the body.

The most immediate concern with DVT is that the clot can break free and travel through the bloodstream to the lungs, where it becomes a **pulmonary embolism (PE)**. A PE can obstruct a pulmonary artery and cause severe damage to the lungs and other organs, which can be fatal without quick medical intervention.

While many people with DVT do not experience any noticeable symptoms, others may experience swelling, pain, or redness in the affected leg. In some cases, the condition can be asymptomatic, which is why regular screening is essential for those at high risk.

Symptoms of DVT

The symptoms of DVT can vary depending on the location and size of the clot. Some people with DVT may have no symptoms at all, making the condition difficult to detect without diagnostic tests. However, when symptoms do occur, they are often related to restricted blood flow and inflammation in the affected area.

Common Symptoms of DVT Include:

- **Swelling**: Swelling in the leg is one of the most common signs of DVT. It may appear suddenly and affect the entire leg or just one area. The affected leg may be noticeably larger than the unaffected leg.
- **Pain or Tenderness**: People with DVT often experience pain or tenderness in the affected leg, especially when walking or standing. The pain may start in the calf and can feel like cramping or soreness.
- **Red or Discolored Skin**: The skin over the clot may appear red or have a bluish tint due to poor circulation. This discoloration is often associated with increased pressure in the veins.
- **Warmth**: The area around the clot may feel warm to the touch due to inflammation in the veins.
- **Swelling in the Arms**: While less common, DVT can also occur in the arms, leading to swelling, discomfort, and possible redness in the affected limb.

Signs of a Pulmonary Embolism (PE)

If a clot breaks loose and travels to the lungs, it can cause a **pulmonary embolism**. Symptoms of a PE include:

- **Sudden Shortness of Breath**: A person may feel short of breath or unable to catch their breath, even when at rest.
- **Chest Pain**: The pain from a PE can feel like a sharp, stabbing sensation in the chest, similar to that of a heart attack.
- **Coughing (with or without blood)**: A person with a PE may cough up blood or have a persistent, dry cough.
- **Rapid Heart Rate**: A PE can cause an elevated heart rate as the body attempts to compensate for the lack of oxygen.
- **Dizziness or Fainting**: If a PE is large, it can lead to a drop in blood pressure, causing dizziness, lightheadedness, or even fainting.

These symptoms are serious and require immediate medical attention. If you or someone you know experiences signs of a PE, seek emergency care right away.

Certain conditions and behaviors increase the risk of developing DVT. Understanding these risk factors can help individuals take proactive steps to prevent the condition.

1. Prolonged Immobility

One of the most significant risk factors for DVT is prolonged immobility. People who are confined to a bed for long periods (such as after surgery, illness, or injury) are at a higher risk of blood clots because they are not moving their muscles, which normally help with blood circulation. Long car trips or airplane flights that require sitting for extended periods also increase the risk.

2. Surgery and Injury

Surgical procedures, particularly those involving the legs, hips, or abdomen, can damage blood vessels and increase the likelihood of clot formation. Similarly, serious injuries to the lower extremities can lead to blood pooling and clotting. Orthopedic surgery, such as hip or knee replacements, carries a particularly high risk.

3. Pregnancy and Postpartum Period

Pregnancy significantly increases the risk of DVT due to hormonal changes and pressure from the growing uterus. During pregnancy, the body's blood clotting mechanisms become more active to prevent excessive bleeding during childbirth. Additionally, women are at heightened risk in the weeks following childbirth.

4. Cancer and Cancer Treatments

Certain cancers, such as those of the pancreas, lungs, and gastrointestinal tract, increase the likelihood of clotting. Additionally, treatments like chemotherapy, which can damage blood vessels and increase clotting factors, further raise the risk of DVT.

5. Obesity

Obesity contributes to DVT in several ways. Excess body weight places added pressure on the veins, especially in the legs, impairing circulation and increasing the likelihood of blood clots. Obesity is also associated with other medical conditions, such as diabetes and high blood pressure, which further increase the risk.

6. Genetic Conditions

Some individuals inherit genetic conditions that make their blood more prone to clotting. These conditions, known as **thrombophilias**, include **Factor V Leiden mutation**, **protein C or S deficiency**, and **antithrombin deficiency**. People with these genetic abnormalities are at a higher risk of DVT and may require additional medical supervision or blood-thinning medications.

7. Hormonal Medications

Hormonal therapies, such as oral contraceptives (birth control pills) or hormone replacement therapy (HRT), increase the risk of blood clots. Estrogen, in particular, can alter the blood's ability to clot, raising the risk of DVT. Women who smoke while taking hormonal medications are at an even greater risk.

8. Age

As individuals age, the risk of developing DVT increases. Older adults are more likely to experience conditions like immobility, cancer, and cardiovascular diseases, which all contribute to the formation of blood clots.

Diagnosis of DVT

The diagnosis of deep vein thrombosis is based on a combination of physical examination, medical history, and diagnostic tests. If DVT is suspected, doctors will typically perform the following:

1. Physical Exam

A doctor will examine the affected leg for signs of swelling, tenderness, redness, and warmth. They may also perform a **Homans' sign test** (though this is not always reliable), which involves gently dorsiflexing the foot to check for calf pain.

2. Ultrasound

Ultrasound is the primary imaging test used to confirm the presence of a blood clot. It uses high-frequency sound waves to create an image of the veins and detect any blockages.

3. D-dimer Test

A **D-dimer test** measures the presence of a substance released when a blood clot breaks down. Elevated D-dimer levels can suggest that a clot may be present, but this test alone is not enough to confirm DVT. It is usually combined with imaging tests.

4. CT Scan or MRI

In certain cases, a **CT scan** or **MRI** may be used to visualize clots in larger veins or to rule out other conditions. These tests are particularly useful for detecting clots in the pelvis or abdominal area.

Prevention of DVT

Preventing deep vein thrombosis is vital, especially for individuals at higher risk. Several lifestyle changes, medical interventions, and precautionary measures can help reduce the risk of DVT.

1. Staying Active

Regular exercise is one of the most effective ways to improve circulation and reduce the risk of DVT. Moving the legs, even in small ways (e.g., flexing the ankles), can help maintain blood flow. For those on long flights or car rides, standing up and walking every hour is recommended.

2. Compression Stockings

For individuals at high risk of DVT, **compression stockings** can help improve blood flow in the legs. These specially designed stockings apply pressure to the legs, reducing swelling and preventing blood from pooling in the veins.

3. Hydration

Staying well-hydrated is essential for maintaining healthy circulation. Dehydration can cause blood to become thicker and more likely to clot, increasing the risk of DVT. Drinking plenty of fluids during travel or while immobile is crucial.

4. Anticoagulant Medications

For those with a history of DVT or other risk factors, **anticoagulants** (blood thinners) may be prescribed to help prevent clot formation. These medications reduce the blood's ability to clot and are often used after surgery or in patients with certain chronic conditions.

5. Early Mobilization After Surgery

After surgery, it is essential to get up and move as soon as possible, provided the healthcare team gives approval. Early mobilization helps stimulate circulation and reduces the risk of DVT.

Conclusion

Deep vein thrombosis is a serious condition that, if left untreated, can lead to potentially life-threatening complications such as pulmonary embolism. Recognizing the symptoms of DVT, understanding the risk factors, and taking proactive measures to prevent clot formation are essential to maintaining health and preventing serious outcomes. By staying active, managing risk factors, and following medical advice, individuals can significantly reduce the likelihood of developing DVT and protect their overall cardiovascular health.

Chapter 25

Anticoagulants and Thrombosis Treatment

Thrombosis, including deep vein thrombosis (DVT) and pulmonary embolism (PE), is a significant medical concern due to the potential for life-threatening complications. A blood clot that forms in a deep vein can travel to the lungs, resulting in a pulmonary embolism, a condition that can quickly become fatal if not diagnosed and treated promptly. One of the primary ways to manage these conditions is through anticoagulant therapy and clot-busting treatments, which aim to either prevent further clot formation or dissolve existing clots. In this chapter, we will explore the different medical treatments used to manage DVT and pulmonary embolism, the mechanisms by which they work, and the important considerations in their use.

What Are Anticoagulants?

Anticoagulants, often referred to as **blood thinners**, are medications designed to prevent blood clotting or **coagulation**. They do not directly dissolve clots but rather interfere with the blood clotting process, reducing the risk of further clot formation. By reducing the blood's ability to form new clots, anticoagulants allow the body's natural fibrinolytic system (which dissolves clots) to work more effectively.

Anticoagulants are commonly used in the treatment and prevention of conditions like DVT, PE, atrial fibrillation, and stroke, among others. There are several different classes of anticoagulants, each with its own mechanisms of action, side effects, and clinical indications.

Types of Anticoagulants

There are two main types of anticoagulants used in the treatment of thrombosis: **oral anticoagulants** and **injectable anticoagulants**. Both types of anticoagulants work to reduce the blood's ability to form clots, but they differ in how they are administered, their side effects, and their required monitoring.

1. Oral Anticoagulants

Oral anticoagulants are taken in pill form and work by inhibiting specific proteins in the blood coagulation cascade that are involved in clot formation. These drugs are usually taken daily and require regular monitoring in some cases.

Warfarin (Coumadin)

Warfarin is one of the oldest and most well-known oral anticoagulants. It works by inhibiting the action of vitamin K, a key element required for clotting factor production in the liver. By reducing the amount of vitamin K available, warfarin decreases the ability of the blood to form clots.

Warfarin has been used for decades to treat DVT and prevent pulmonary embolism. However, it requires frequent blood tests (called **INR tests**) to monitor the drug's effects and adjust the dosage accordingly. Warfarin's effectiveness can be influenced by diet (particularly foods rich in vitamin K, such as leafy greens) and certain medications, making careful management crucial.

Direct Oral Anticoagulants (DOACs)

More recently, **direct oral anticoagulants (DOACs)** have become a popular alternative to warfarin due to their ease of use and lower need for monitoring. DOACs work by targeting specific coagulation factors rather than affecting vitamin K. They are taken in a single daily dose and do not require routine blood tests to monitor their effect. Some common DOACs include:

- **Dabigatran (Pradaxa)**: Inhibits thrombin, a critical enzyme in the clotting process.
- **Rivaroxaban (Xarelto), Apixaban (Eliquis)**, and **Edoxaban (Savaysa)**: These drugs target factor Xa, an enzyme that plays a role in clot formation.

DOACs have been shown to be just as effective as warfarin in preventing blood clots but with fewer dietary restrictions and a lower risk of bleeding complications. However, unlike warfarin, these medications do not have a readily available antidote for reversing their effects in the event of serious bleeding, although research into reversal agents for DOACs is ongoing.

2. Injectable Anticoagulants

Injectable anticoagulants are typically administered in a hospital or clinical setting. These drugs are used for acute treatment of thrombosis, especially when immediate anticoagulation is necessary. Injectable anticoagulants work by targeting specific steps in the clotting cascade, either by inhibiting thrombin or factor Xa.

Heparin

Heparin is one of the most commonly used injectable anticoagulants. It works by enhancing the activity of **antithrombin**, a protein in the blood that inactivates clotting factors, particularly **factor Xa** and **thrombin**. By binding to antithrombin, heparin accelerates its ability to prevent clot formation.

Heparin is often used in emergency situations, such as when a patient is first diagnosed with DVT or PE. It is typically given intravenously in the hospital and closely monitored through blood tests to ensure the correct dosage. Low-molecular-weight heparins (LMWH), such as **enoxaparin (Lovenox)**, are a more refined form of heparin that can be administered as an injection under the skin (subcutaneously) and are often used for outpatient care.

Fondaparinux (Arixtra)

Fondaparinux is a synthetic anticoagulant that works similarly to heparin but targets **factor Xa** more specifically. It is used in the treatment of DVT and PE and is given by injection. Fondaparinux is often used in patients who have experienced a clotting episode and need immediate anticoagulation. Like LMWH, it is used for short-term treatment, with oral anticoagulants typically being introduced once the acute phase has passed.

Clot-Busting Drugs: Thrombolytics

In addition to anticoagulants, another important class of drugs used in the treatment of thrombosis is **thrombolytics** or **fibrinolytics**. These drugs are used to dissolve clots directly, rather than merely preventing their formation. Thrombolytic therapy is typically reserved for cases where a clot has caused severe complications, such as a massive PE or a stroke.

Thrombolytic medications work by activating the body's natural fibrinolytic system, which breaks down fibrin, a protein that helps form the structure of a clot. The most common thrombolytic drugs include:

- **Alteplase (Activase)**: A tissue plasminogen activator (tPA) that helps break down fibrin and dissolve clots.
- **Streptokinase**: A thrombolytic agent derived from bacteria, although less commonly used today due to the risk of allergic reactions.

Thrombolytics are typically administered intravenously in a hospital setting, and the treatment carries a significant risk of bleeding. Due to the potential for serious bleeding complications, thrombolytic therapy is generally reserved for cases where the clot is life-threatening and other treatments are insufficient.

When Are Anticoagulants and Thrombolytics Used?

The choice between anticoagulant therapy and thrombolytic therapy depends on the severity of the condition, the location of the clot, and the patient's overall health.

Acute Management of DVT and PE

In the case of an acute DVT or PE diagnosis, the first line of treatment typically involves the use of injectable anticoagulants (e.g., heparin or LMWH) to immediately reduce the risk of further clotting. Once the patient is stabilized, they may be transitioned to an oral anticoagulant (e.g., warfarin or a DOAC) for long-term management and to prevent the formation of new clots.

In some cases, such as with a massive PE, where there is a high risk of death or organ damage, thrombolytic therapy may be considered. The decision to use thrombolytics is based on the severity of the PE, the patient's overall health, and the potential risks involved.

Prevention of DVT and PE Recurrence

Patients who have experienced a DVT or PE episode are typically placed on long-term anticoagulation therapy to prevent the recurrence of clots. The duration of anticoagulant treatment depends on the underlying cause of the clot and the patient's risk factors. For example, individuals with a first-time DVT may need to be on anticoagulants for a few months, while those with ongoing risk factors, such as cancer, may require lifelong anticoagulation.

Surgical Intervention

In rare cases, when anticoagulants or thrombolytics are not effective, or when there is a contraindication to their use, surgical interventions may be necessary. These interventions may include the insertion of a **vena cava filter (IVC filter)**, a small device placed in the large vein (inferior vena cava) that helps prevent clots from traveling to the lungs. In more extreme cases, **surgical thrombectomy** may be performed to remove the clot.

Side Effects and Risks of Anticoagulant and Thrombolytic Therapy

While anticoagulants and thrombolytics are critical in the treatment of thrombosis, they come with risks, primarily related to bleeding. Because these medications interfere with the body's ability to form clots, they increase the likelihood of bleeding complications, especially in individuals with certain conditions (e.g., recent surgery, gastrointestinal ulcers, or liver disease).

Common side effects of anticoagulants and thrombolytics include:

- **Excessive bleeding**: Uncontrolled or prolonged bleeding from cuts, bruising, or internal bleeding.
- **Nosebleeds and gum bleeding**: These are more common with certain anticoagulants, such as warfarin or DOACs.
- **Bruising**: Patients taking anticoagulants may notice that they bruise more easily.
- **Allergic reactions**: Some patients may experience allergic reactions to certain thrombolytic drugs.

To minimize the risk of bleeding complications, patients on anticoagulants must be closely monitored. Regular blood tests, such as **INR tests** for warfarin and kidney function tests for DOACs, are essential to ensure the drugs are working properly without increasing the risk of bleeding. Additionally, patients are often instructed to avoid activities that could lead to injury, such as contact sports, while undergoing treatment.

Conclusion

Anticoagulants and thrombolytics play a crucial role in the treatment of thrombosis, including DVT and pulmonary embolism. These medications help prevent clot formation and, in the case of thrombolytics, actively dissolve existing clots. While they are life-saving treatments, they require careful monitoring and management to minimize the risk of bleeding complications. Early detection of DVT or PE, prompt initiation of treatment, and adherence to medical recommendations are key factors in improving outcomes and preventing serious complications.

Chapter 26

Genetic Factors and Thrombophilia

Thrombosis, the formation of abnormal blood clots in veins and arteries, is a significant health concern that can lead to life-threatening conditions like deep vein thrombosis (DVT) and pulmonary embolism (PE). While environmental and lifestyle factors play a crucial role in the development of blood clots, there is also a genetic component that can increase a person's susceptibility to clotting disorders. This chapter will explore how genetics influence the risk of developing thrombophilia—a condition where the blood has an increased tendency to clot— and the implications of genetic factors in the diagnosis, prevention, and treatment of thrombosis.

What Is Thrombophilia?

Thrombophilia refers to a group of disorders that predispose individuals to an increased risk of developing abnormal blood clots. In a healthy circulatory system, the blood maintains a delicate balance between coagulation (clotting) and fibrinolysis (clot breakdown). When this balance is disrupted, either due to excessive clotting or insufficient breakdown, blood clots can form in veins and arteries, leading to conditions such as DVT, PE, or stroke.

There are two main types of thrombophilia:

1. **Inherited Thrombophilia**: Caused by genetic mutations or abnormalities that lead to a higher tendency for blood to clot.
2. **Acquired Thrombophilia**: Resulting from other factors such as pregnancy, hormonal therapy, certain cancers, or prolonged immobility.

Inherited thrombophilia is the focus of this chapter, and it can be passed down through generations, leading to a family history of clotting disorders. Genetic mutations related to thrombophilia can affect various components of the coagulation system, including proteins that regulate clot formation and breakdown. These genetic factors can make individuals more susceptible to developing abnormal blood clots, sometimes even in the absence of other risk factors.

The Role of Genetics in Thrombophilia

Genetics plays a pivotal role in the development of thrombophilia by influencing how the body's clotting system functions. Some individuals inherit mutations in genes that affect proteins involved in the coagulation process. These genetic mutations may result in an overactive clotting system, where the blood forms clots too easily or does not dissolve clots efficiently.

The following genetic mutations are most commonly associated with inherited thrombophilia:

1. Factor V Leiden Mutation

One of the most well-known genetic mutations related to thrombophilia is the **Factor V Leiden** mutation. Factor V is a protein that plays a critical role in the blood clotting cascade. The mutation in the factor V gene leads to a protein that is resistant to inactivation by activated protein C, an anticoagulant protein that helps regulate clotting. This resistance causes an increased risk of clot formation, especially in the veins, leading to conditions such as DVT and PE.

Factor V Leiden is the most common inherited thrombophilia, affecting approximately 5% of people of European descent. Individuals with one copy of the mutation (heterozygous) have a two to four times higher risk of developing clots, while those with two copies (homozygous) have an even greater risk, up to 80 times higher.

2. Prothrombin Gene Mutation (G20210A)

Another genetic mutation associated with increased clotting risk is the **prothrombin gene mutation**, also known as **G20210A**. Prothrombin is a clotting factor that, when activated, converts to thrombin, a key enzyme in the clotting process. The G20210A mutation leads to elevated levels of prothrombin in the blood, increasing the likelihood of clot formation.

Individuals with the prothrombin gene mutation have a higher risk of developing venous thrombosis, particularly in the lower legs (DVT) or the lungs (PE). The mutation is less common than Factor V Leiden but still significant, with an estimated prevalence of 2-3% in the general population, particularly among individuals of European descent.

3. Protein C and Protein S Deficiencies

Protein C and protein S are natural anticoagulants in the blood that help prevent excessive clotting by inactivating clotting factors like Factor V and Factor VIII. Inherited deficiencies of these proteins can increase the risk of venous thromboembolism (VTE), a condition where blood clots form in veins and can travel to the lungs, causing PE.

- **Protein C Deficiency**: Individuals with protein C deficiency have a reduced ability to inhibit clot formation. This condition is inherited in an autosomal dominant pattern, meaning that inheriting just one copy of the mutated gene can lead to a higher risk of clots. This deficiency can be present from birth, and in severe cases, it can cause life-threatening clotting events in childhood.
- **Protein S Deficiency**: Similar to protein C deficiency, protein S deficiency results in an inability to properly regulate clotting. Protein S acts as a cofactor to protein C, enhancing its ability to inactivate clotting factors. A deficiency in protein S leads to an increased risk of thrombosis, and like protein C deficiency, it can be inherited in an autosomal dominant pattern.

Both protein C and protein S deficiencies are relatively rare, but they are significant risk factors for developing DVT and PE, particularly in individuals with a family history of clotting disorders.

4. Antithrombin III Deficiency

Antithrombin III (ATIII) is another natural anticoagulant that helps to control clot formation by inhibiting clotting factors such as thrombin and Factor Xa. A deficiency in ATIII increases the likelihood of developing blood clots, particularly in the veins.

Antithrombin III deficiency can be inherited or acquired, but when it is inherited, it is often passed down in an autosomal dominant pattern. Individuals with this deficiency have an increased risk of developing thrombosis, and they may require lifelong anticoagulation therapy to prevent clots. ATIII deficiency is rare, but it is an important consideration in the diagnosis and management of inherited thrombophilia.

5. Homocysteine Levels and MTHFR Gene Mutations

Elevated homocysteine levels in the blood (known as **hyperhomocysteinemia**) are associated with an increased risk of clotting disorders. Homocysteine is an amino acid that, when present in high levels, can damage blood vessels and increase the risk of clot formation.

Genetic mutations in the **MTHFR gene** (methylenetetrahydrofolate reductase) are linked to elevated homocysteine levels. MTHFR is responsible for converting homocysteine into other amino acids, and mutations in this gene can impair this process, leading to increased homocysteine levels in the blood.

Though hyperhomocysteinemia alone is not always sufficient to cause thrombosis, it can act as a contributing factor in individuals who have other genetic risk factors, such as Factor V Leiden or protein C deficiency. Elevated homocysteine levels can often be managed with vitamin B12, B6, and folate supplementation, which help to lower homocysteine levels and reduce clotting risk.

Inheritance Patterns of Thrombophilia

Inherited thrombophilia is typically passed down through families according to **autosomal dominant** inheritance patterns. This means that an individual only needs to inherit one copy of the mutated gene from one parent to have an increased risk of developing thrombosis.

However, having a genetic mutation does not guarantee that an individual will develop a clot. Environmental factors, such as prolonged immobility, smoking, hormonal therapy, and pregnancy, can all interact with genetic predispositions to increase the risk of clotting. Many people with genetic mutations associated with thrombophilia live without ever experiencing a clotting event, while others may face multiple occurrences over the course of their lives.

Genetic Testing for Thrombophilia

Genetic testing for thrombophilia can help identify individuals who are at higher risk of developing blood clots. Testing is typically recommended for individuals with a personal or family history of unexplained blood clots, particularly if these clots occurred at a young age or in unusual circumstances, such as during pregnancy or after surgery.

Genetic tests can detect mutations in genes related to Factor V Leiden, prothrombin, protein C and S deficiencies, antithrombin III deficiency, and other clotting disorders. However, it is important to understand that genetic testing for thrombophilia is not always recommended for everyone, as it may not alter the course of treatment for individuals who have not experienced clotting events. Moreover, the results of genetic testing should be interpreted in the context of the individual's clinical history and other risk factors.

Management and Treatment of Thrombophilia

For individuals diagnosed with inherited thrombophilia, the primary goal is to reduce the risk of thrombosis. This may include:

- **Anticoagulant therapy**: Long-term use of blood thinners like warfarin, heparin, or DOACs to reduce the risk of clot formation.
- **Lifestyle modifications**: Avoiding prolonged periods of immobility, maintaining a healthy weight, quitting smoking, and managing other risk factors such as high blood pressure and diabetes.
- **Monitoring during high-risk situations**: Pregnant women or those undergoing surgery may require careful monitoring and anticoagulation management to reduce the risk of blood clots.

In cases where thrombophilia leads to a clotting event, immediate treatment with anticoagulants is necessary to prevent further complications. Additionally, people with thrombophilia should work closely with healthcare providers to develop a personalized treatment plan based on their genetic risk and medical history.

Conclusion

Genetic factors play a significant role in the development of thrombophilia and the risk of abnormal blood clot formation. Inherited mutations in genes associated with clotting factors such as Factor V Leiden, prothrombin, protein C, protein S, and antithrombin III contribute to an increased likelihood of developing thrombosis. By understanding the genetic basis of thrombophilia, healthcare providers can offer more personalized prevention and treatment strategies to reduce the risk of life-threatening blood clots. As genetic testing and research continue to advance, our understanding of thrombophilia will help shape more effective management and intervention approaches, allowing individuals with inherited clotting disorders to lead healthier lives.

Chapter 27

Risk Factors for Blood Clots: Lifestyle and Environmental Considerations

Blood clots are a serious medical condition that can have life-threatening consequences, including deep vein thrombosis (DVT) and pulmonary embolism (PE). While genetic factors and underlying health conditions play a significant role in the development of these clotting disorders, lifestyle and environmental factors also contribute to the risk. This chapter will explore the key lifestyle and environmental risk factors that can increase the likelihood of developing blood clots, including obesity, smoking, prolonged immobility, and other considerations, and how individuals can take steps to minimize their risk.

The Basics of Blood Clots

Blood clots are essential to the body's natural healing process, helping to stop bleeding when we get injured. However, when blood clots form abnormally, especially inside veins or arteries without a clear injury to the blood vessels, they can lead to dangerous health problems. Clots that form in the deep veins of the legs are called **deep vein thrombosis (DVT)**, while those that break free and travel to the lungs are known as **pulmonary embolism (PE)**.

DVT occurs when a blood clot forms in a deep vein, typically in the legs or pelvis, and can cause swelling, pain, and redness. When part of the clot breaks off and travels through the bloodstream to the lungs, it can block a pulmonary artery, resulting in PE. PE is a medical emergency that can cause severe breathing difficulties and even death.

While some individuals may be genetically predisposed to forming blood clots, lifestyle and environmental factors can significantly influence the likelihood of developing these conditions. Understanding these risk factors is crucial for prevention and reducing the overall burden of clot-related health issues.

Obesity: A Major Contributor to Blood Clotting Risk

One of the most significant lifestyle factors influencing the risk of developing blood clots is **obesity**. Obesity is characterized by excessive body fat, and it is a major risk factor for numerous chronic diseases, including cardiovascular disease, diabetes, and hypertension. Additionally, obesity has a direct impact on the circulatory system and can contribute to the development of blood clots in several ways:

Increased Pressure on Veins

Obesity increases the pressure on veins, especially in the lower legs. The excess weight can lead to poor circulation and reduce the efficiency of the venous system, which is responsible for returning blood to the heart. This poor circulation can make it more difficult for the body to clear clots and increase the risk of DVT. Over time, this can lead to the formation of clots in the veins, which can migrate to the lungs and cause PE.

Higher Levels of Inflammation

Obesity is also associated with chronic low-grade inflammation in the body, which contributes to the development of clotting. Adipose tissue (body fat) secretes pro-inflammatory cytokines, which can activate clotting factors in the blood. These inflammatory molecules can increase the likelihood of clot formation and make it more difficult for the body to resolve clots once they form.

Hormonal Changes

In obese individuals, hormonal changes related to excess body fat can further increase the risk of blood clots. For example, obesity is linked to increased levels of estrogen, which can promote clotting. Women who are obese and also use birth control pills or hormone replacement therapy (HRT) are at a heightened risk for developing clotting disorders due to the combined effects of hormones and excess weight.

Smoking: The Detrimental Effects on the Circulatory System

Smoking is another major lifestyle factor that significantly increases the risk of developing blood clots. The chemicals in cigarette smoke have a toxic effect on the blood vessels and blood cells, which can make the blood more prone to clotting.

Damage to Blood Vessels

Smoking leads to damage to the endothelial lining of blood vessels, which is crucial for maintaining proper blood flow. When the endothelium is damaged, it triggers the body's clotting mechanisms to try to heal the blood vessel. This can result in the formation of blood clots that could potentially lead to DVT or PE.

Increased Blood Coagulation

Smoking has also been shown to increase blood viscosity (thickness), which can make blood flow less efficiently through the circulatory system. Thicker blood is more likely to form clots, particularly in veins. Moreover, smoking has been linked to the activation of clotting factors, which makes the blood more prone to coagulation.

Interaction with Other Risk Factors

The risk of developing blood clots is compounded when smoking is combined with other risk factors, such as obesity or prolonged immobility. For example, smokers who are overweight or sedentary have a higher risk of DVT and PE compared to individuals who maintain a healthy weight and are non-smokers.

Prolonged Immobility: A Hidden Danger to Circulation

Prolonged **immobility** is one of the most significant environmental risk factors for developing blood clots. When a person remains in one position for an extended period, such as during long flights, hospital stays, or recovery from surgery, the blood flow in the legs can become sluggish, which increases the risk of clot formation. This is commonly referred to as **venous stasis**, and it is a key contributor to DVT.

The Impact of Long-Distance Travel

Extended periods of immobility are often associated with **long-distance travel**, particularly air travel. Passengers sitting for hours in cramped seats during long flights are at risk of developing DVT, a condition commonly referred to as "economy class syndrome." The limited space in the seats and the inability to move around regularly causes blood to pool in the veins, especially in the legs, creating an environment where clots can easily form.

Hospitalization and Surgery

Hospitalization, especially following surgery, is another common situation where immobility increases the risk of clotting. Surgical procedures, particularly those involving the lower limbs or abdomen, can cause trauma to the blood vessels and disrupt normal blood flow. Combined with the immobility often required during the recovery process, this makes patients more susceptible to developing blood clots. In these situations, doctors may recommend the use of **compression stockings** or **anticoagulant medications** to reduce the risk of DVT.

The Role of Physical Activity

Physical activity plays a critical role in maintaining healthy circulation. Regular movement helps to keep the blood flowing efficiently, reducing the likelihood of blood pooling in the veins. Individuals who lead sedentary lifestyles, especially those who spend long hours sitting or lying down, should make efforts to stand, stretch, and walk around periodically to stimulate blood flow and reduce the risk of clot formation.

Other Environmental and Lifestyle Risk Factors

In addition to obesity, smoking, and immobility, there are several other environmental and lifestyle factors that can increase the risk of blood clots:

Hormonal Contraception and Pregnancy

Women who use hormonal contraception (such as birth control pills, patches, or rings) are at a higher risk of developing blood clots, especially if they smoke or are overweight. Pregnancy itself also increases the risk of clot formation due to hormonal changes, increased blood volume, and pressure on the veins from the growing uterus.

Age and Gender

While not entirely lifestyle-related, **age** and **gender** can influence clotting risk. The risk of DVT and PE increases with age, particularly after age 60, due to changes in blood vessel health and circulation. Additionally, women are more likely than men to develop blood clots, especially during pregnancy, the postpartum period, and while using hormonal contraceptives.

Chronic Medical Conditions

Chronic medical conditions such as **heart disease**, **diabetes**, and **cancer** can contribute to an increased risk of blood clots. People with these conditions often have impaired circulation or altered blood properties that can make clotting more likely. Medications used to treat these conditions, such as hormone therapy or certain chemotherapy drugs, can further elevate the risk.

Prevention and Lifestyle Modifications

Preventing blood clots involves making healthy lifestyle choices and minimizing environmental risk factors. Here are some strategies for reducing the risk of DVT and PE:

- **Maintain a Healthy Weight**: Regular physical activity and a balanced diet can help you achieve and maintain a healthy weight, reducing the pressure on your veins and lowering your risk of clotting.
- **Quit Smoking**: Giving up smoking can improve blood vessel health, reduce inflammation, and decrease the likelihood of clot formation.
- **Stay Active**: Regular exercise helps maintain good circulation and reduces the risk of venous stasis. Aim for at least 150 minutes of moderate-intensity exercise per week.
- **Move During Long Trips**: If you're traveling for long periods, take breaks to stand, stretch, and walk around. Consider wearing compression stockings to support your circulation.
- **Manage Chronic Conditions**: If you have a chronic condition like heart disease, diabetes, or obesity, work with your doctor to manage it effectively and reduce the associated clotting risks.

Conclusion

Lifestyle and environmental factors play a significant role in the development of blood clots, and understanding these risks can help individuals take proactive steps to protect their health. Obesity, smoking, and prolonged immobility are some of the primary contributors to clot formation, but by making healthier lifestyle choices, individuals can reduce their risk. Regular physical activity, maintaining a healthy weight, quitting smoking, and staying vigilant during long periods of immobility are key strategies for preventing blood clots and their potentially life-threatening complications. By taking these steps, individuals can safeguard their circulatory health and reduce the burden of conditions like deep vein thrombosis and pulmonary embolism.

Chapter 28

Prevention and Early Intervention: The Key to Managing Thrombosis

Blood clots are a common health concern that can lead to serious complications, such as deep vein thrombosis (DVT) and pulmonary embolism (PE). While blood clotting is a necessary function of the body to stop bleeding after an injury, the formation of clots inappropriately within blood vessels can cause life-threatening conditions. Prevention and early intervention are crucial in managing thrombosis and mitigating the risks associated with it. Through simple yet effective lifestyle changes, such as exercise, a healthy diet, and mindful lifestyle practices, individuals can reduce their risk of blood clot formation and improve overall circulatory health. This chapter will provide a comprehensive guide to preventing blood clots, focusing on the importance of exercise, dietary choices, and other habits that contribute to vascular well-being.

The Role of Prevention and Early Intervention

Prevention is the cornerstone of managing thrombosis. For those at risk, whether due to a medical condition, a genetic predisposition, or external factors like surgery or immobility, proactive measures can dramatically reduce the chances of blood clot development. Recognizing the early warning signs of thrombosis and responding quickly is equally important in preventing serious outcomes. Early intervention, including medical treatments such as blood thinners and clot-busting medications, can stop clots from growing and traveling, which reduces the risk of complications like PE.

The primary causes of thrombosis are related to stasis of blood flow, changes in the blood's composition (increased clotting tendency), and damage to the blood vessels. When blood flow slows down, particularly in veins, the blood is more likely to pool and form clots. Factors like sedentary behavior, obesity, and smoking can contribute to blood stagnation. Likewise, inflammation and other medical conditions, such as cancer and pregnancy, can also alter the blood's clotting factors. Through lifestyle adjustments, individuals can help ensure that their blood remains fluid and their circulation stays efficient.

Exercise: Vital for Circulatory Health

One of the most effective ways to prevent blood clots is regular physical activity. Exercise not only strengthens the heart and lungs, but it also promotes healthy circulation, which is crucial for preventing clots. The muscles, especially those in the legs, assist in pumping blood back to the heart, and regular movement keeps the blood flowing freely throughout the body.

When you engage in physical activity, you activate your muscles, which helps to keep the blood moving through veins, particularly in the legs. This is especially important for individuals who are at a higher risk of DVT due to prolonged periods of immobility, such as during long flights or extended bed rest. It is also essential for those with a sedentary lifestyle. Maintaining a regular exercise routine helps to prevent the blood from pooling in the lower extremities and encourages overall cardiovascular health.

Exercise has an additional benefit in its ability to reduce inflammation in the body. Chronic inflammation is a known contributor to the development of blood clots. By lowering the levels of inflammation through consistent physical activity, you can also decrease the likelihood of clot formation.

Regular exercise helps to maintain a healthy weight, and obesity is a well-established risk factor for thrombosis. Excess weight puts added strain on the veins, particularly in the lower body, and can hinder proper blood flow. Exercise helps to manage weight by burning calories, increasing muscle mass, and improving metabolism, all of which contribute to a reduced risk of clots.

A wide range of physical activities can benefit circulatory health, including walking, cycling, swimming, and strength training. For those who are new to exercise or have mobility issues, low-impact activities like yoga or gentle stretching can also be incredibly effective in promoting healthy blood flow. Aiming for at least 150 minutes of moderate-intensity exercise per week can dramatically improve vascular health.

Dietary Choices: Fueling Your Body to Prevent Clots

Diet plays a pivotal role in thrombosis prevention. Certain nutrients are known to help prevent blood clots by improving circulation and reducing inflammation, while others can contribute to an increased risk of clotting. A diet rich in whole foods, such as fruits, vegetables, lean proteins, and healthy fats, can help protect the body from clotting disorders.

Foods high in **omega-3 fatty acids** are especially beneficial for reducing the risk of clotting. Omega-3s, found in fatty fish-like salmon, mackerel, and sardines, as well as flaxseeds and walnuts, have anticoagulant properties that help to keep the blood from becoming too thick and sticky. These healthy fats also reduce inflammation, which is a contributing factor in clot formation. Including omega-3-rich foods in your diet can help maintain smooth and efficient circulation.

Antioxidants, found in colorful fruits and vegetables, are another crucial part of a clot-preventing diet. Berries, spinach, kale, and other antioxidant-rich foods help neutralize free radicals in the body, which can damage blood vessels and promote clotting. By fighting oxidative stress, antioxidants help maintain the integrity of blood vessels and prevent the buildup of substances that could lead to clot formation.

Garlic is a well-known natural blood thinner and offers multiple cardiovascular benefits. It contains allicin, a compound that has been shown to help reduce blood viscosity, making it less likely for clots to form. Incorporating garlic into your meals not only enhances flavor but also supports the circulatory system.

Turmeric and **ginger**, two common spices, have anti-inflammatory properties that help reduce the likelihood of blood clot formation. Curcumin, the active compound in turmeric, has been shown to reduce blood clotting by interfering with certain clotting factors. Similarly, ginger contains gingerol, which inhibits clot formation and promotes healthy circulation. These spices can be easily added to your diet through smoothies, teas, or cooked dishes.

Staying hydrated is another essential component of preventing blood clots. Dehydration causes the blood to become thicker, which increases the likelihood of clotting. Drinking adequate amounts of water daily helps keep the blood at a proper viscosity, making it easier for the circulatory system to function effectively. In addition to water, herbal teas and water-rich foods like fruits and vegetables also contribute to hydration.

While there are many foods that can help prevent clots, it's also important to be mindful of those that can increase clotting risk. **Trans fats**, found in processed foods and fried items, contribute to inflammation and can lead to higher clotting tendencies. Similarly, an overconsumption of **refined sugars** and **carbohydrates** can lead to obesity, insulin resistance, and chronic inflammation, all of which are risk factors for clotting disorders. It's essential to minimize the intake of these foods in favor of more wholesome, nutrient-dense options.

Lifestyle Adjustments: Small Changes for Big Impact

In addition to diet and exercise, several other lifestyle changes can help prevent blood clots. One of the most significant changes is **quitting smoking**. Smoking is a major risk factor for thrombosis, as it damages blood vessels and increases blood clotting. The chemicals in tobacco promote inflammation and disrupt the normal function of blood cells and vessels, increasing the likelihood of clots. If you smoke, seeking help to quit can significantly reduce your risk of developing dangerous clots.

Maintaining a healthy **weight** is another key factor in reducing the risk of blood clots. Obesity places extra stress on the veins, particularly in the lower body, and increases the risk of clotting. Losing excess weight through a combination of exercise and healthy eating helps to alleviate this pressure and improves circulation. Even modest weight loss can make a significant difference in reducing the risk of thrombosis.

For individuals who spend long periods sitting or standing, such as during long flights or desk jobs, taking breaks to **move around** is essential. **Elevating the legs**, **stretching**, and **walking** periodically can help prevent blood from pooling in the veins and reduce the likelihood of clot formation. For people at high risk, wearing **compression stockings** can also help support circulation and prevent blood from accumulating in the legs.

Medical Interventions for High-Risk Individuals

In cases where lifestyle changes alone are not enough, or if an individual is at an especially high risk for thrombosis, medical interventions may be necessary. **Anticoagulants**, commonly known as blood thinners, are prescribed to reduce the risk of clot formation. These medications help prevent the blood from becoming too thick and help to maintain smooth, unimpeded circulation. Regular medical check-ups are necessary to monitor the effectiveness of these treatments and ensure the patient's safety.

For those who have had a previous blood clot, **compression devices** or **medications** may be recommended to prevent further clotting episodes. In some instances, **clot-busting medications** or surgical interventions may be required if a clot has formed, posing an immediate threat to health.

Recognizing the Signs of Thrombosis

Recognizing the symptoms of blood clots is crucial for early intervention. Common symptoms of **DVT** include **swelling, pain or tenderness** in one leg, and **redness** or **warmth** in the affected area. **Pulmonary embolism** symptoms include **shortness of breath, chest pain, rapid heart rate**, and **coughing up blood**. If any of these symptoms occur, it is essential to seek immediate medical attention to prevent severe complications.

Conclusion

Prevention and early intervention are the most effective ways to manage the risk of thrombosis. Through consistent exercise, a diet rich in blood-thinning and anti-inflammatory foods, and lifestyle changes such as quitting smoking and maintaining a healthy weight, individuals can significantly reduce the likelihood of developing blood clots. By taking proactive steps to promote healthy circulation and recognizing the warning signs of clots, we can protect ourselves from the potentially dangerous consequences of thrombosis. By implementing these strategies, thrombosis can be managed effectively, ensuring long-term vascular health and well-being.

Chapter 29

The Role of Stem Cells in Blood Disorders

Stem cell therapies have emerged as a groundbreaking development in the medical field, offering hope for the treatment of a range of blood disorders, including sickle cell anemia, leukemia, and other hematologic conditions. The potential of stem cells to regenerate and repair damaged tissue, including blood cells, has transformed the way medical professionals approach these diseases. Stem cell treatments offer not only a chance to alleviate symptoms but, in some cases, a potential cure for conditions that were once considered chronic and incurable. This chapter explores the science behind stem cells, how they are used in treating blood disorders, and the current advancements that are shaping the future of hematologic care.

Understanding Stem Cells: The Building Blocks of Regeneration

Stem cells are unique cells that have the ability to develop into many different types of cells in the body. They possess the remarkable ability to divide and differentiate into specialized cells, making them essential for growth, repair, and regeneration. Stem cells are categorized into two broad types: **embryonic stem cells** and **adult stem cells**. Embryonic stem cells have the ability to form all the cell types in the body, while adult stem cells, found in various tissues, are responsible for the maintenance and repair of those tissues.

The most widely used stem cells in the treatment of blood disorders are **hematopoietic stem cells (HSCs)**. These stem cells are responsible for the production of all the components of blood, including red blood cells, white blood cells, and platelets. Hematopoietic stem cells are found in the bone marrow, which is the body's blood cell factory. They can be harvested and transplanted into patients to treat a variety of blood diseases. By replacing the patient's defective or diseased blood cells with healthy, donor-derived hematopoietic stem cells, doctors can provide patients with a fresh start for their hematologic health.

Stem Cell Transplantation: A Lifeline for Blood Disorders

Stem cell transplantation, also known as a **bone marrow transplant (BMT)**, is one of the most widely used therapies for blood disorders. The process involves the infusion of healthy stem cells into a patient's bloodstream to replace damaged or dysfunctional bone marrow. This therapy is particularly effective for patients with **leukemia, lymphoma,** and **aplastic anemia,** as well as inherited blood disorders like **sickle cell anemia** and **thalassemia.**

In the case of **leukemia,** a type of blood cancer, the bone marrow becomes infiltrated with malignant cells, preventing the production of healthy blood cells. A stem cell transplant helps to restore normal hematopoiesis, giving the patient the opportunity for remission and long-term survival. For patients with **sickle cell anemia,** where abnormal hemoglobin leads to deformed red blood cells that block blood flow, a stem cell transplant offers a potential cure by replacing the defective blood cells with healthy, donor-derived cells. The success of these treatments has transformed the prognosis for many patients, turning previously fatal conditions into manageable diseases.

There are two main types of stem cell transplants: **autologous** and **allogeneic.** In an **autologous transplant,** the patient's own stem cells are harvested, treated, and then reintroduced into the body. This approach is typically used for diseases like certain types of leukemia, where the patient's immune system is not severely compromised. In an **allogeneic transplant,** stem cells are sourced from a donor, often a family member or an unrelated individual who matches the patient's genetic markers. This type of transplant is commonly used for inherited blood disorders, including sickle cell anemia and thalassemia.

Advancements in Stem Cell Therapy for Blood Disorders

Over the past few decades, stem cell research has seen significant advances, especially in the treatment of blood disorders. The development of **gene therapy** and improvements in **stem cell harvesting techniques** have expanded the potential for stem cell therapies to be more effective and widely accessible. **Gene editing technologies,** like **CRISPR-Cas9,** have shown promise in correcting genetic defects at the molecular level, offering a potential cure for conditions like sickle cell anemia and thalassemia without the need for a stem cell transplant. This revolutionary technique allows scientists to modify a patient's own stem cells, correcting the genetic mutation that causes the disorder before reintroducing them into the patient's body. This approach has the potential to reduce the need for donor matches and lower the risk of rejection, offering patients a more personalized and less invasive treatment option.

One of the challenges in stem cell therapy has been the risk of **graft-versus-host disease (GVHD)** in allogeneic transplants. GVHD occurs when the donor's immune cells attack the recipient's tissues, causing inflammation and organ damage. However, recent advances in immunosuppressive therapies and better matching of donors to recipients have significantly reduced the incidence of GVHD, improving the success rate of stem cell transplants.

The Promise of Cord Blood Stem Cells

In addition to traditional bone marrow-derived stem cells, **cord blood** has emerged as an alternative source of hematopoietic stem cells. Cord blood is rich in stem cells and can be collected at the time of birth, offering a potentially life-saving resource for patients in need of a stem cell transplant. Since cord blood stem cells are more "naive" than adult stem cells, they have a lower risk of causing GVHD and may be an excellent option for patients without a matched donor. The growing use of cord blood banks, where donated cord blood is stored for future use, has greatly expanded access to stem cell transplants, offering hope to patients with blood cancers and genetic blood disorders.

Challenges and Future Directions

Despite the promising potential of stem cell therapies, there are still several challenges to overcome. One of the major hurdles is the availability of suitable **donors**. In many cases, finding a genetically matched donor for an allogeneic stem cell transplant can be difficult, especially for patients from minority or underrepresented populations. Efforts are underway to improve stem cell matching techniques and increase the diversity of stem cell donor registries to ensure that all patients have access to life-saving treatments.

Another challenge lies in the **cost** of stem cell therapies. While the potential benefits of stem cell transplants are profound, the cost of these treatments can be prohibitive, especially when factoring in the need for post-transplant care, long-term monitoring, and immunosuppressive medications. However, as stem cell research advances and becomes more widespread, the hope is that the cost of these therapies will decrease, making them more accessible to a broader range of patients.

Despite these challenges, the future of stem cell therapy in blood disorders is incredibly promising. The use of stem cells to treat hematologic conditions is rapidly evolving, with **clinical trials** continually exploring new ways to improve outcomes and reduce risks. Emerging technologies, such as **induced pluripotent stem cells (iPSCs)**, which are adult cells reprogrammed to become stem cells, could revolutionize the treatment of blood disorders by creating a virtually limitless source of stem cells for patients.

Patient Stories and Successes

For many individuals living with sickle cell anemia, leukemia, and other serious blood disorders, stem cell therapy has been nothing short of transformative. Patients who once faced grim prognoses have regained their health and quality of life after undergoing stem cell transplants. These stories of recovery and hope underscore the importance of continued investment in stem cell research and the potential for further breakthroughs.

In particular, children born with genetic blood disorders like sickle cell anemia and thalassemia have benefited from stem cell transplants that have given them a chance at a normal, healthy life. The availability of stem cell-based treatments has significantly improved their long-term survival rates, and many are now able to live without the chronic pain and complications that once dominated their lives.

Conclusion

Stem cell therapies have revolutionized the treatment of blood disorders, offering life-saving solutions to patients with conditions that were once considered intractable. Whether through bone marrow transplants, gene therapy, or the use of cord blood, stem cells have the potential to cure, treat, and significantly improve the lives of those living with blood disorders. As research continues to advance, the future holds great promise for the development of even more effective, less invasive, and widely accessible stem cell treatments. For patients and families affected by blood disorders, these advances represent not just new treatment options, but a new hope for a healthier, more vibrant future.

Chapter 30

Genetic Testing: The Future of Blood Disorder Diagnosis

The field of medicine is evolving rapidly, and one of the most promising areas of growth is genetic testing. By examining a person's genetic makeup, we can better understand their predisposition to certain diseases, including blood disorders. For many years, physicians have relied on traditional diagnostic methods, such as blood tests and imaging, to identify and treat illnesses. However, with advances in **genetic screening** and the development of **personalized medicine**, doctors are now able to detect blood disorders at their earliest stages, predict the risks for certain conditions, and tailor treatments based on an individual's genetic profile. This chapter explores the critical role that genetic testing plays in diagnosing blood disorders and how it is shaping the future of patient care.

The Basics of Genetic Testing

Genetic testing involves analyzing a person's DNA to identify variations or mutations that could be linked to disease. This testing can be used to diagnose existing conditions, predict the likelihood of future diseases, and provide insights into how a person will respond to various treatments. Genetic tests are conducted by extracting DNA from a sample of blood, saliva, or other tissue. This DNA is then sequenced, and scientists look for specific genetic markers or mutations that are associated with particular diseases.

In the context of blood disorders, genetic testing can offer profound benefits. Many blood disorders, such as **sickle cell anemia**, **thalassemia**, **hemophilia**, and **blood cancers** like **leukemia**, have a genetic basis. By understanding these genetic factors, doctors can provide more accurate diagnoses, initiate earlier interventions, and offer personalized treatment plans that are better suited to the patient's unique genetic makeup.

Genetic Testing in Hematology: Unlocking the Mysteries of Blood Disorders

Blood disorders can result from mutations in various genes that affect the production or function of blood cells, clotting factors, or other components of the circulatory system. Understanding the genetics behind these conditions has become increasingly important in diagnosing and treating patients more effectively. Here are a few examples of how genetic testing has made a significant impact:

1. **Sickle Cell Anemia and Thalassemia**: Both sickle cell anemia and thalassemia are caused by inherited genetic mutations that affect hemoglobin, the protein in red blood cells responsible for transporting oxygen throughout the body. Genetic testing allows for the identification of carriers of these mutations and can help diagnose these conditions in newborns or individuals showing symptoms. Early diagnosis is crucial, as it allows for interventions that can improve the quality of life and, in some cases, offer potential cures through stem cell transplants.
2. **Hemophilia**: Hemophilia, a bleeding disorder that prevents blood from clotting properly, is caused by mutations in genes related to clotting factors. Through genetic testing, doctors can determine whether a patient carries the gene for hemophilia, enabling early detection in infants and providing a clearer path for treatment options. Moreover, genetic screening helps determine the severity of the condition, which is critical for managing symptoms and choosing the most appropriate therapies.
3. **Leukemia and Blood Cancers**: Leukemias and other blood cancers arise from mutations in the bone marrow's blood-forming cells. Certain genetic mutations, such as those in the **BCR-ABL** gene (common in chronic myelogenous leukemia), can be detected through genetic testing. Identifying these mutations enables doctors to diagnose the specific type of leukemia and tailor treatment, such as targeted therapies that block the effects of the mutated gene. In addition, genetic testing can provide information on the likelihood of remission, recurrence, and response to chemotherapy or other treatments.
4. **Inherited Platelet Disorders**: Platelet disorders, which affect blood clotting and can lead to conditions like **thrombocytopenia** or excessive bleeding, can also be identified through genetic testing. Mutations in genes responsible for platelet production or function can be detected, providing early warnings for individuals at risk of bleeding complications. Genetic screening can guide treatment options such as platelet transfusions or drugs to help manage clotting.

Personalized Medicine: Tailoring Treatments to the Individual

One of the most exciting advancements in genetic testing is the rise of **personalized medicine**, which uses an individual's genetic profile to determine the most effective treatments. In the case of blood disorders, this approach means that treatments can be tailored not only to the specific condition a person has but also to the way their body will respond to various therapies.

For instance, **genetic variations** in enzymes responsible for drug metabolism can affect how well a person responds to medications. Through genetic testing, doctors can identify these variations and select the most effective medications or adjust dosages to avoid side effects or ineffective treatments. For patients with blood cancers like leukemia, genetic testing can identify mutations that make the disease resistant to certain drugs. As a result, doctors can prescribe **targeted therapies**, which are designed to block the specific mutation that is driving the cancer, offering more precise and effective treatment options.

In addition to providing more effective treatments, genetic testing in personalized medicine also reduces the trial-and-error approach to treatment. Instead of relying on broad-based therapies that might not be suitable for everyone, genetic testing ensures that patients receive the most optimal care based on their unique genetic makeup. This approach not only improves patient outcomes but can also reduce healthcare costs by minimizing ineffective treatments and hospitalizations.

Preconception and Prenatal Genetic Testing

Genetic testing is not limited to the diagnosis and treatment of blood disorders once they are present. **Preconception genetic screening** allows individuals or couples to test for inherited blood disorders before pregnancy. For example, individuals who are carriers of sickle cell anemia or thalassemia can use genetic testing to assess the likelihood of passing these conditions on to their children. This allows prospective parents to make informed decisions and, if necessary, seek medical advice or consider options such as **in vitro fertilization (IVF)** with genetic screening to avoid having a child with a blood disorder.

Additionally, prenatal genetic testing can detect blood disorders in a fetus. By performing non-invasive procedures, such as testing maternal blood or amniotic fluid, doctors can identify genetic mutations linked to blood disorders like **hemophilia** or **sickle cell disease** early in the pregnancy. Early diagnosis allows for better management of the disease, including potential treatments or interventions before birth.

Ethical Considerations and Challenges

While the benefits of genetic testing in blood disorder diagnosis and treatment are clear, there are also important ethical considerations. For example, the information gathered through genetic testing could impact an individual's privacy and could potentially be misused by employers or insurance companies. Laws such as the **Genetic Information Nondiscrimination Act (GINA)** in the United States have been put in place to protect against such misuse, but ethical concerns still remain about the potential for discrimination based on genetic information.

Moreover, genetic testing can sometimes present difficult choices. For instance, when a family learns that their child carries the gene for a serious blood disorder, such as sickle cell anemia, they may face emotional and psychological challenges in deciding how to proceed with prenatal testing, treatment options, or family planning. These decisions are deeply personal and often require counseling and guidance from healthcare professionals.

The Future of Genetic Testing and Blood Disorders

Looking forward, the field of genetic testing is rapidly evolving, and the future promises even more exciting developments. **Next-generation sequencing** technology, which allows for faster and more accurate genetic testing, is becoming increasingly accessible, meaning that more patients will be able to benefit from early and precise diagnosis of blood disorders.

Additionally, the combination of **genetic testing** with **artificial intelligence (AI)** and **machine learning** could revolutionize how doctors interpret genetic data. AI algorithms have the potential to analyze vast amounts of genetic information to predict the likelihood of developing certain blood disorders, recommend treatment plans, and even identify previously overlooked patterns in disease genetics. These technologies could significantly enhance the accuracy of diagnoses and the effectiveness of treatments.

In terms of **gene therapy**, which aims to correct the genetic mutations causing blood disorders, genetic testing will play a pivotal role in identifying the specific mutations that need to be targeted. Advances in **CRISPR-Cas9** gene-editing technology may one day allow doctors to precisely alter the DNA of patients with blood disorders, potentially curing them of their conditions altogether.

Conclusion

Genetic testing has become a cornerstone of modern medicine, particularly in the diagnosis and treatment of blood disorders. From identifying inherited genetic mutations that cause conditions like sickle cell anemia and hemophilia to guiding personalized treatment plans, genetic testing has transformed the landscape of hematology. As technology continues to evolve, genetic screening and personalized medicine will play an even greater role in improving outcomes for patients with blood disorders, offering hope for more effective treatments, earlier diagnoses, and even potential cures. The future of blood disorder diagnosis and management is increasingly intertwined with genetics, and with ongoing advancements, we are poised to make significant strides in the fight against these debilitating diseases.

Chapter 31

Advances in Blood Transfusion Medicine

Blood transfusions have been a cornerstone of medical treatment for over a century, saving millions of lives every year. From trauma victims to patients undergoing surgery, those suffering from blood disorders, and even those needing routine treatments like chemotherapy, blood transfusions play an essential role in modern medicine. However, like all medical procedures, blood transfusion carries risks, including infections, allergic reactions, and transfusion-related complications. Over the years, researchers and medical professionals have worked tirelessly to improve the safety, efficacy, and efficiency of blood transfusions. With advances in technology and scientific understanding, the field of transfusion medicine is evolving rapidly, making the process safer and more reliable than ever before.

The History and Necessity of Blood Transfusions

The practice of blood transfusion dates back to the early 17th century, but it wasn't until the early 20th century that major breakthroughs in blood typing and compatibility allowed for transfusions to be performed safely. Before the discovery of blood types, transfusions often resulted in disastrous outcomes. However, once **Karl Landsteiner** discovered the different blood types (A, B, AB, and O), the risk of complications was significantly reduced, opening the door to widespread transfusion practices.

Today, transfusions are used to treat a variety of conditions, such as severe blood loss from trauma or surgery, **anemia**, **hemophilia**, and other blood disorders. The basic principle behind blood transfusion is straightforward: replacing a person's lost or deficient blood components with donor blood. However, the complexity of ensuring compatibility between the donor's blood and the recipient's blood has led to continuous advancements in the field.

Blood Screening: Ensuring Safety through Testing

One of the most important improvements in blood transfusion safety has been the development of comprehensive blood screening techniques. Before blood is transfused, it undergoes rigorous testing to ensure that it is free from infectious agents, such as **HIV**, **hepatitis B and C**, **syphilis**, and **malaria**. These infections can be transmitted through contaminated blood, and modern screening methods are designed to detect these pathogens with high precision and reliability.

The use of **nucleic acid testing (NAT)** is one such advancement that has revolutionized blood safety. NAT technology allows for the detection of viruses in the blood at much earlier stages than traditional methods, dramatically reducing the window period during which a viral infection could go undetected. This has greatly minimized the risk of transmitting diseases through blood transfusions, ensuring that the blood supply remains safe for patients worldwide.

In addition to infectious disease testing, blood typing and crossmatching remain critical components of ensuring transfusion safety. Compatibility between a donor's and recipient's blood type is essential, and more sophisticated testing has allowed for better matching, reducing the risk of hemolytic reactions and other adverse outcomes.

Blood Conservation Technologies

While blood transfusions are often a lifesaving intervention, they are not without risks. Because of this, there has been significant focus on developing blood conservation strategies that reduce the need for transfusions altogether. These strategies aim to minimize the use of donated blood and ensure that it is available for those who need it most.

Cell-salvage technology is one such advancement that has proven particularly useful in surgeries involving significant blood loss. Cell salvage works by collecting blood lost during surgery, washing it, and then returning it to the patient's body. This process ensures that the patient receives their own blood, eliminating the risk of incompatibility or transmission of infectious agents.

In addition, **erythropoietin (EPO),** a hormone that stimulates the production of red blood cells, has been used in preoperative settings to boost a patient's red blood cell count and reduce the need for transfusion. The use of EPO, often in combination with iron supplementation, has helped patients undergoing major surgeries, especially those at high risk of anemia, to maintain their red blood cell levels, thus decreasing reliance on donor blood.

For patients with chronic conditions such as **anemia** or **chronic kidney disease**, **iron therapy** and other hematopoietic agents are increasingly being used to help the body produce more red blood cells, which can help alleviate the need for frequent transfusions. This shift toward blood conservation technologies is an essential step in ensuring that blood products are available when needed most, particularly in times of blood shortages or in regions with limited access to blood donation programs.

Advanced Blood Component Therapy

Blood is not a single fluid, but a complex mixture of components, including **red blood cells (RBCs), white blood cells (WBCs), platelets**, and **plasma**. In recent years, the ability to separate and transfuse specific blood components has revolutionized transfusion medicine. Today, rather than administering whole blood, patients receive the precise component they need.

- **Red Blood Cell Transfusions**: The most common use of blood transfusions is to restore the levels of red blood cells, particularly in cases of anemia or blood loss. Advances in **leukoreduction**—the process of removing white blood cells from blood products—have reduced the risk of febrile reactions and alloimmunization, a process in which a patient develops antibodies against transfused blood. This ensures a more effective and safe transfusion.
- **Platelet Transfusions**: Platelet transfusions are often necessary for patients with bleeding disorders or those undergoing chemotherapy. New technologies, such as **pheresis**, allow for the selective collection of platelets from donors, which can then be used to help patients with low platelet counts. Moreover, ongoing research into **platelet storage** techniques continues to extend the shelf-life of platelets, making them more readily available when needed.
- **Plasma Transfusions**: Plasma is a yellowish liquid that contains water, electrolytes, proteins, and waste products. It is used to treat patients with clotting disorders or burns. Advances in plasma fractionation techniques have made it possible to isolate and purify clotting factors from plasma, which can then be used in **hemophilia** treatments, significantly improving patient outcomes.

Blood Substitutes: The Quest for Synthetic Blood

One of the most exciting areas of transfusion medicine is the development of **blood substitutes**—synthetic or artificial blood products designed to perform the functions of human blood. Although researchers have been working on blood substitutes for decades, challenges remain in replicating the complex properties of natural blood. Still, progress continues to be made, and blood substitutes hold promise for treating trauma patients, those with rare blood types, or people in areas where access to blood donations is limited.

Two primary types of blood substitutes are being researched:

- **Hemoglobin-based oxygen carriers (HBOCs)**: These are artificial molecules designed to carry oxygen, much like natural hemoglobin. They are derived from purified hemoglobin, often extracted from outdated blood donations or produced synthetically. HBOCs can be stored longer than whole blood, making them an appealing option in emergencies or in settings where blood storage is a challenge.
- **Perfluorocarbon (PFC)-based blood substitutes**: PFCs are synthetic compounds that can dissolve large amounts of oxygen. While not yet in widespread use, PFCs have shown promise in animal studies and early human trials. They are capable of carrying oxygen throughout the body and can be used in cases of severe blood loss where traditional blood transfusions are not immediately available.

Despite their potential, blood substitutes are not yet a viable alternative to human blood, and much more research is needed to refine these technologies. However, they represent an exciting frontier in transfusion medicine, with the potential to reduce the dependency on blood donations and provide life-saving treatments in emergency situations.

The Role of Artificial Intelligence and Data in Blood Transfusion

In recent years, **artificial intelligence (AI)** and **machine learning** have begun to play an increasing role in transfusion medicine. These technologies are being used to predict blood demand, match blood donors with recipients more efficiently, and even assess the safety and compatibility of blood products. AI-driven algorithms can analyze large datasets from blood banks to help predict the number of donations needed during emergencies, ensuring that blood products are available when and where they are needed most.

AI is also being used to track and monitor transfusion reactions, providing real-time data that can help clinicians intervene early in case of complications. This can lead to better management of transfusions and minimize adverse reactions, further improving patient safety.

The Future of Blood Transfusion Medicine

As technology continues to advance, the future of blood transfusion medicine looks promising. Innovations in blood component therapy, blood conservation strategies, and the development of blood substitutes will continue to improve patient outcomes. Moreover, AI and data analytics will enhance the precision of transfusion practices, ensuring that blood products are used more efficiently and safely.

While challenges remain, especially in ensuring a safe and adequate blood supply, the progress made in transfusion medicine is undeniable. Blood transfusions will continue to play a crucial role in modern healthcare, saving lives and improving patient outcomes. As the field evolves, the ultimate goal will be to make blood transfusions as safe, accessible, and effective as possible, bringing us closer to a future where life-saving treatments are available to everyone, everywhere.

Chapter 32

Bone Marrow Transplants: A Life-Saving Procedure

Bone marrow transplants (BMT) have become a cornerstone in the treatment of several life-threatening diseases, including leukemia, lymphoma, and severe anemia. This medical procedure offers a last-resort treatment option for patients whose bone marrow is no longer capable of producing healthy blood cells. Although it can be a complex and risky process, the advancements in stem cell research, tissue matching, and post-transplant care have made bone marrow transplants a more accessible and effective treatment for a variety of blood disorders.

What is Bone Marrow?

Bone marrow is a soft, spongy tissue located in the center of certain bones, such as the pelvis, spine, ribs, and sternum. It is the body's blood cell factory, producing red blood cells, white blood cells, and platelets. These blood cells are critical for oxygen transport, immune defense, and clotting functions. Bone marrow produces millions of blood cells each day, maintaining a delicate balance to meet the body's needs.

When a patient's bone marrow becomes damaged or defective, as seen in conditions like **leukemia**, **lymphoma**, **aplastic anemia**, and some inherited blood disorders, it can no longer produce these cells in sufficient quantity or quality. Bone marrow failure can lead to dangerous complications, such as **anemia**, **infections**, and **excessive bleeding**. In these cases, a bone marrow transplant offers a potential cure by replacing the damaged or diseased marrow with healthy marrow from a donor.

What is a Bone Marrow Transplant?

A bone marrow transplant, also known as **hematopoietic stem cell transplantation (HSCT)**, involves replacing the defective bone marrow with healthy stem cells, which are the progenitor cells that can develop into all types of blood cells. There are two main types of bone marrow transplants:

1. **Autologous Transplant**: In this type of transplant, the patient's own stem cells are collected, often before they undergo chemotherapy or radiation

therapy. These cells are then reintroduced into the patient's body after their original, diseased marrow has been destroyed. Autologous transplants are typically used for diseases like **multiple myeloma** and certain types of **lymphoma**.

2. **Allogeneic Transplant**: This type involves using stem cells from a genetically matched donor. The donor may be a relative, such as a sibling, or an unrelated individual who has a compatible tissue type. Allogeneic transplants are more complex and carry greater risks but are often used for diseases such as **leukemia**, **aplastic anemia**, and **myelodysplastic syndromes**.

The Process of Bone Marrow Transplantation

The process of a bone marrow transplant can be broken down into several key stages: **pre-transplant evaluation**, **conditioning**, **the transplant itself**, and **post-transplant care**.

- **Pre-Transplant Evaluation**: Before undergoing a bone marrow transplant, patients undergo extensive testing to assess their overall health, suitability for the procedure, and the compatibility of the donor's stem cells. This evaluation includes blood tests, imaging studies, and assessments of the heart, lungs, and other organs. The patient's medical history and any underlying conditions are also reviewed to minimize complications during the procedure.
- **Conditioning**: Prior to the transplant, patients undergo a process called conditioning, which typically involves chemotherapy and/or radiation. The purpose of conditioning is to destroy the patient's diseased bone marrow and suppress their immune system to prevent rejection of the transplanted stem cells. While conditioning is essential for the success of the transplant, it also comes with significant risks, including weakened immunity, infections, and damage to healthy tissues.
- **The Transplant**: The actual transplant involves infusing the patient with healthy stem cells via an intravenous (IV) line, similar to a blood transfusion. If the patient is receiving an **autologous transplant**, their previously harvested stem cells are reintroduced. For an **allogeneic transplant**, the donor's stem cells are infused. The transplanted stem cells travel to the bone marrow, where they begin to produce new blood cells. This is referred to as engraftment, and it typically occurs within two to four weeks after the transplant.

- **Post-Transplant Care**: After the transplant, the patient's immune system is very weak, and they are highly susceptible to infections. Post-transplant care includes rigorous monitoring, frequent blood tests, medications to prevent infections, and drugs to manage any side effects from the conditioning regimen. Over time, the patient's new immune system begins to strengthen, and they gradually recover from the transplant.

Complications and Risks of Bone Marrow Transplants

While bone marrow transplants can be life-saving, they come with risks and potential complications. Some of the most common risks associated with BMT include:

- **Graft-Versus-Host Disease (GVHD)**: In an **allogeneic transplant**, the transplanted immune cells from the donor can recognize the patient's body as foreign and attack it, a condition known as graft-versus-host disease. GVHD can range from mild to severe and can affect the skin, liver, and gastrointestinal tract. Chronic GVHD can significantly impact the patient's quality of life and require long-term immunosuppressive treatment.
- **Infections**: Since the patient's immune system is severely compromised following the transplant, infections are a major concern. Both bacterial and viral infections can be life-threatening if not quickly diagnosed and treated. Patients are placed on prophylactic antibiotics and antiviral drugs to help prevent infections, but careful monitoring is essential.
- **Engraftment Failure**: In some cases, the transplanted stem cells fail to engraft, meaning they do not establish themselves in the patient's bone marrow. This can result in a failure to produce new blood cells, which can lead to prolonged anemia, bleeding, and infections. In some cases, a second transplant may be necessary.
- **Organ Damage**: Chemotherapy and radiation used during the conditioning phase can cause damage to vital organs such as the heart, liver, and lungs. The risk of organ damage is increased in older patients or those with pre-existing health conditions. Organ function is closely monitored after transplant to detect any signs of damage.

Success Rates and Prognosis

The success of a bone marrow transplant depends on a variety of factors, including the type of disease being treated, the age and overall health of the patient, the compatibility of the donor, and how well the patient responds to treatment. For diseases like leukemia and lymphoma, bone marrow transplants can offer a potential cure, with some patients experiencing long-term remission. In cases of severe anemia or inherited blood disorders like **thalassemia**, bone marrow transplants can improve quality of life by eliminating the need for regular blood transfusions.

In general, younger patients tend to fare better than older patients, and those who receive a transplant at an earlier stage of their disease often experience better outcomes. Advances in **HLA matching** (human leukocyte antigen matching) have also increased the likelihood of finding compatible donors, thereby improving success rates in allogeneic transplants.

Advances in Bone Marrow Transplant Technology

The field of bone marrow transplantation has seen significant improvements in recent years, driven by advances in medical technology, stem cell research, and genetic science. Some of the most promising advancements include:

- **Stem Cell Collection and Processing**: New techniques for harvesting and processing stem cells have made the procedure safer and more effective. For example, **peripheral blood stem cell (PBSC) collection** allows doctors to collect stem cells from the bloodstream instead of directly from the bone marrow. This method is less invasive, more comfortable for the donor, and results in higher numbers of stem cells for the transplant.
- **Improved HLA Matching**: The development of more precise tissue typing techniques has made it easier to find a donor with a close match. Better matching reduces the risk of rejection and complications like GVHD. Some research is focused on using stem cells from **umbilical cord blood** or **induced pluripotent stem cells (iPSCs)** to create more universally compatible sources of stem cells.
- **Gene Therapy**: Researchers are exploring the use of **gene editing technologies** like **CRISPR-Cas9** to correct genetic defects in a patient's own stem cells before transplanting them. This could be a game-changer for patients with inherited blood disorders, such as **sickle cell disease** and **thalassemia**, as it could provide a more personalized and effective treatment.
- **Reduced Intensity Conditioning**: Advances in **reduced intensity conditioning (RIC)** have made bone marrow transplants an option for older patients or those with other health problems. RIC uses lower doses of

chemotherapy and radiation, reducing the strain on the patient's body while still allowing the transplanted cells to engraft and function.

The Future of Bone Marrow Transplants

As research into stem cell therapies and transplant techniques continues, the future of bone marrow transplantation looks increasingly promising. With ongoing advancements in genetics, immunology, and cell-based therapies, we may soon see more effective treatments for blood cancers, inherited blood disorders, and other conditions. While the procedure remains complex and challenging, the potential for life-saving outcomes and long-term remission is greater than ever. Bone marrow transplants represent a vital part of the medical landscape, offering hope for patients with conditions that once seemed intractable.

Through the continued evolution of this field, the dream of curing blood disorders and improving the lives of patients undergoing these procedures is slowly becoming a reality, offering a future where bone marrow transplants could become even more successful, less invasive, and accessible to all those who need them.

Chapter 33

Targeted Therapies and New Drugs for Blood Disorders

The landscape of medicine is continuously evolving, especially in the realm of blood disorders. Over the past few decades, medical research has ushered in a new era of treatment through **targeted therapies** and **novel drug options**. These advancements have significantly improved the way blood-related diseases, including **leukemia, lymphoma, sickle cell anemia**, and **hemophilia**, are managed, offering patients more effective treatments with fewer side effects. This chapter will explore how emerging drug treatments and targeted therapies are transforming the management of blood disorders, focusing on their mechanisms, the conditions they treat, and their impact on patients' lives.

Understanding Targeted Therapy

Targeted therapy refers to a class of treatments that specifically target the molecular mechanisms driving disease. Unlike traditional therapies, such as chemotherapy, which attack rapidly dividing cells indiscriminately, targeted therapies are designed to disrupt the specific molecules involved in the growth and survival of diseased cells. This precision offers the potential for greater efficacy and fewer side effects, as healthy cells are less affected.

In blood disorders, particularly blood cancers like **leukemia and lymphoma**, the use of targeted therapies has revolutionized treatment protocols. These drugs often target specific proteins, enzymes, or genetic mutations within cancerous cells that allow them to proliferate uncontrollably. By blocking these molecular pathways, targeted therapies can stop the growth of cancer cells, induce cell death, and reduce the need for more aggressive treatments like chemotherapy and radiation.

Targeted Therapies in Hematologic Malignancies

Blood cancers, including **acute leukemia, chronic leukemia, lymphoma**, and **myeloma**, often rely on **targeted therapies** to provide more effective, less toxic treatments. Several classes of drugs have been developed to target the mutations and biological processes specific to these cancers:

- **Tyrosine Kinase Inhibitors (TKIs)**: One of the most widely known and utilized types of targeted therapy in hematologic malignancies are **TKIs**. These drugs block the action of enzymes called tyrosine kinases, which are involved in the signaling pathways that allow cancer cells to grow and divide. **Imatinib** (Gleevec), for example, is a TKI used to treat **chronic myelogenous leukemia (CML)**. It specifically targets the BCR-ABL fusion protein, which is present in most cases of CML and plays a key role in the cancer's development. TKIs have dramatically improved survival rates for CML patients and are considered a standard of care for this condition.
- **Monoclonal Antibodies**: These lab-created antibodies are designed to target specific proteins on the surface of cancer cells. For example, **rituximab** is a monoclonal antibody used in the treatment of **non-Hodgkin lymphoma**. It targets a protein called CD20, which is found on the surface of B-cells, the type of white blood cells affected by lymphoma. By binding to CD20, rituximab triggers the immune system to destroy the lymphoma cells.
- **Proteasome Inhibitors**: In the treatment of **multiple myeloma**, a cancer of plasma cells, drugs like **bortezomib** (Velcade) inhibit the proteasome, a cellular structure that degrades unwanted proteins. By blocking this process, proteasome inhibitors accumulate damaged proteins inside the cancerous cells, leading to cell death. These drugs have proven to be effective in extending survival and improving the quality of life for patients with multiple myeloma.

Emerging Drug Treatments for Sickle Cell Disease

While the development of **targeted therapies** has been instrumental in blood cancers, advances are also being made for **non-cancerous blood disorders** such as **sickle cell disease** (SCD). SCD is an inherited blood disorder where the red blood cells become crescent-shaped, leading to blockages in blood vessels, pain, and organ damage. Traditional treatments for sickle cell disease, including blood transfusions and pain management, do not address the root cause of the disorder.

However, a new wave of **genetic therapies** and **drug treatments** are offering hope for SCD patients:

- **Hydroxyurea**: Hydroxyurea is a drug that has been used for years to reduce the frequency of pain crises and other complications in SCD patients. It works by stimulating the production of fetal hemoglobin (HbF), a type of hemoglobin that is more effective at carrying oxygen and helps prevent the sickling of red blood cells. While it does not cure sickle cell disease, hydroxyurea has been shown to significantly improve quality of life and reduce hospitalizations for many patients.

- **Gene Therapy**: Perhaps the most exciting development in the treatment of sickle cell disease is **gene therapy**. This emerging treatment aims to correct the genetic mutation responsible for sickle cell disease by either replacing the faulty gene or reactivating the production of fetal hemoglobin. The treatment involves harvesting a patient's own stem cells, editing the genes in a lab, and then transplanting them back into the patient's body. This approach has shown promise in clinical trials, offering the potential for a permanent cure for sickle cell disease.

- **Voxelotor**: A newer drug, **Voxelotor** (Oxbryta), was approved by the FDA for the treatment of sickle cell disease. This drug works by increasing the affinity of hemoglobin for oxygen, preventing the sickling of red blood cells and improving overall oxygen delivery to tissues. Voxelotor has shown significant improvements in hemoglobin levels and has been a breakthrough in managing the disease, especially for those who do not respond well to traditional treatments like hydroxyurea.

- **Crizanlizumab**: Another FDA-approved treatment for sickle cell disease is **Crizanlizumab** (Adakveo), a monoclonal antibody that works by preventing the adhesion of sickled cells to blood vessel walls, thereby reducing pain crises. This drug has been shown to decrease the frequency of vaso-occlusive crises (pain episodes) in SCD patients, significantly improving their quality of life.

Gene Editing: The Next Frontier in Blood Disorder Treatment

As genetic understanding of blood disorders continues to improve, **gene editing technologies** such as **CRISPR-Cas9** hold immense promise for treating a variety of blood-related conditions. These tools allow scientists to directly modify the DNA within a patient's cells, offering a new approach to cure genetic disorders at their root.

In sickle cell disease, **CRISPR** has been used to edit the hemoglobin gene, either by correcting the mutation responsible for sickling or by reactivating fetal hemoglobin production. The first clinical trials using CRISPR to treat sickle cell disease have yielded encouraging results, with some patients achieving normal or near-normal hemoglobin levels following treatment. While these therapies are still in the experimental stage, they represent the future of personalized, precision medicine for blood disorders.

Beyond sickle cell disease, **gene editing** holds potential for treating other inherited blood disorders, such as **thalassemia, hemophilia**, and **beta-thalassemia**. In the case of hemophilia, where the body lacks functional clotting factors, gene therapies that introduce the correct genes to produce these factors have been developed. Several clinical trials are currently underway, and the possibility of long-term treatment or even a cure for hemophilia is becoming a realistic goal.

The Impact of New Drugs on Patients' Lives

The advent of **targeted therapies** and **novel drug treatments** has had a profound impact on the lives of patients with blood disorders. For those with blood cancers, the ability to target specific proteins and mutations has led to better treatment outcomes, fewer side effects, and a higher quality of life. Drugs like **tyrosine kinase inhibitors** and **monoclonal antibodies** have allowed many patients to experience long-term remissions, allowing them to return to normal, healthy lives after years of treatment.

For patients with **non-cancerous blood disorders** such as sickle cell disease, new drugs and gene therapies are providing relief from debilitating symptoms, reducing hospital visits, and offering the hope of a cure. **Hydroxyurea, Voxelotor**, and **Crizanlizumab** have transformed the management of sickle cell disease, making it easier for patients to lead active lives.

Perhaps most importantly, the development of **gene therapies** and **gene editing** holds the potential to revolutionize treatment for blood disorders by offering permanent cures. With advances in **personalized medicine**, where treatments are tailored to the genetic makeup of individual patients, the future of blood disorder treatment looks incredibly promising. The ability to offer cures rather than just symptom management could significantly alter the trajectory of many patients' lives, offering them the chance to live without the burden of chronic disease.

Conclusion

The field of blood disorder treatment has undergone remarkable advancements over the past few decades, with **targeted therapies**, **gene therapies**, and **novel drug treatments** playing a pivotal role in transforming patient outcomes. These therapies are not only providing more effective treatment options but are also improving the overall quality of life for patients who once had limited choices. As research continues to progress, we can expect even more breakthroughs in the treatment of blood disorders, leading to greater hope and better outcomes for individuals affected by these conditions. Whether through gene editing, personalized drugs, or stem cell therapies, the future of blood disorder management looks brighter than ever.

Chapter 34

Coping with Chronic Illness: Mental Health Challenges

Living with a chronic blood disorder is more than just a physical battle. It is a psychological and emotional journey that affects patients and their families in profound ways. Chronic conditions such as **sickle cell disease**, **hemophilia**, **thalassemia**, and **blood cancers** often require lifelong management, numerous medical treatments, and ongoing challenges. These conditions not only alter the physical health of those affected but can also lead to significant mental health struggles that impact every aspect of life. This chapter explores the **mental health challenges** associated with chronic blood disorders, the emotional toll on patients and their families, and strategies for coping and managing these challenges.

The Psychological Toll of Chronic Illness

The diagnosis of a blood disorder can be overwhelming. For many patients, the onset of symptoms is sudden and unexplained, often leading to a sense of confusion, fear, and helplessness. Once a diagnosis is made, patients are typically faced with a lifelong journey of managing their condition, which can bring a range of emotional challenges.

One of the most common emotional responses to living with a chronic illness is **anxiety**. Patients often worry about the future, wondering whether their condition will worsen or how they will cope with the ongoing symptoms. For example, individuals with **sickle cell disease** may live in constant fear of painful episodes, known as sickle cell crises, or the risk of organ damage that can result from the condition. Similarly, those with **hemophilia** may experience anxiety about the risk of bleeding and the possibility of serious injury, leading to a hypervigilant approach to daily life.

The **uncertainty** of chronic blood disorders often fuels feelings of helplessness. Patients may experience a loss of control over their own bodies, as symptoms can be unpredictable and difficult to manage. Over time, this lack of control can lead to feelings of frustration and hopelessness, particularly for those with conditions like **chronic myelogenous leukemia** (CML) or **myelodysplastic syndromes** (MDS), where the prognosis may vary, and treatment regimens can be lengthy and grueling.

Another emotional challenge often faced by individuals with blood disorders is **depression**. The impact of managing a chronic illness, combined with physical symptoms and lifestyle adjustments, can be mentally exhausting. Patients with **thalassemia** or **sickle cell disease**, for instance, often undergo frequent hospital visits, blood transfusions, and long periods of pain, which can lead to a sense of isolation. The constant cycle of treatments, medications, and hospitalizations can contribute to **burnout**, a feeling of emotional exhaustion that makes it harder for individuals to maintain a positive outlook.

Additionally, the social stigma associated with certain blood disorders can exacerbate mental health issues. Diseases such as **hemophilia** and **sickle cell disease** have often been misunderstood by the public, leading to misperceptions and discriminatory attitudes. For example, patients with sickle cell disease may be viewed as weak or lazy due to the fatigue associated with the condition, while individuals with hemophilia may feel isolated because their condition is invisible to others unless they experience an episode. This stigma can lead to feelings of **shame** and **social alienation**, further contributing to anxiety and depression.

The Emotional Impact on Families

The emotional toll of living with a blood disorder does not only affect the patient but also has a profound impact on their family members and caregivers. Parents of children with chronic blood disorders such as **thalassemia** or **hemophilia** often face the anxiety of watching their child endure medical procedures and the fear of complications. The emotional burden on caregivers is particularly intense, as they are responsible for managing the patient's medical care, which may include administering medications, organizing doctor visits, and ensuring that the patient is following the prescribed treatment plan.

For families of patients with **blood cancers**, the stress can be compounded by the uncertainty of prognosis and the intensity of treatment. **Chemotherapy, radiation**, and **bone marrow transplants** are often part of the treatment regimens, and these therapies can take a significant emotional toll on both patients and their loved ones. The stress of watching a loved one go through harsh treatments, sometimes with debilitating side effects, can create feelings of **helplessness** and **grief**. In some cases, families may experience **caregiver burnout**, a state of emotional exhaustion and frustration from the constant responsibility of caregiving, which can strain family relationships.

The emotional stress experienced by family members can also affect the dynamics of family life. For example, siblings of children with blood disorders may feel neglected, as much of the attention may be focused on the patient. **Social isolation** is a common concern for families, as dealing with a chronic illness can limit opportunities for socializing, travel, or family activities. This isolation can deepen feelings of frustration and **resentment** within the family, which in turn can exacerbate the emotional burden on everyone involved.

Coping Strategies for Patients and Families

While the mental health challenges associated with chronic blood disorders are real and often debilitating, there are various coping strategies that can help patients and their families navigate the emotional impact of these conditions. A combination of **psychological support**, **peer support**, **education**, and **self-care** can empower patients and families to manage their emotional health and improve their quality of life.

One of the most effective ways to cope with the psychological challenges of chronic illness is through **psychotherapy. Cognitive-behavioral therapy (CBT)** is particularly beneficial for patients with blood disorders, as it helps them reframe negative thoughts, manage anxiety, and develop healthier coping mechanisms. Therapy can provide a safe space for patients to express their emotions, process the psychological impact of their illness, and learn stress-management techniques. **Family therapy** can also be invaluable for helping family members cope with the emotional strain of caregiving and improve communication and support systems within the household.

Another powerful tool for managing the mental health challenges of chronic illness is the establishment of a strong **support network**. Support groups, both in-person and online, can connect patients with others who are living with similar conditions. Sharing experiences and challenges with people who truly understand can reduce feelings of isolation and provide a sense of solidarity. Support groups offer patients and families a chance to share coping strategies, resources, and emotional support in a nonjudgmental environment.

Peer support from others who have experienced the same condition can also play a pivotal role in providing comfort and advice. Many patients find strength in hearing from others who have successfully navigated the challenges of their illness and treatment. These connections offer hope, encouragement, and a sense of community that can be incredibly valuable in reducing stress and anxiety.

Patients with blood disorders can also benefit from **mindfulness** and **relaxation techniques** such as meditation, yoga, or deep breathing exercises. These practices help reduce stress and improve overall mental health by promoting a sense of calm and relaxation. **Mindfulness-based stress reduction (MBSR)** is a technique that has been shown to decrease symptoms of anxiety and depression, improve emotional regulation, and help patients manage the stress associated with chronic illness.

Maintaining a **healthy lifestyle** is another important strategy for coping with the emotional impact of blood disorders. Regular physical activity, a balanced diet, and adequate sleep can all improve mood, reduce stress, and increase overall well-being. Patients who engage in physical exercise often experience a reduction in feelings of depression and anxiety, as exercise stimulates the release of endorphins, the body's natural mood elevators.

The Role of Advocacy and Education

Education and advocacy are essential in managing the emotional and social impact of blood disorders. Raising awareness about these conditions can help reduce **stigmatization** and **misunderstanding**, allowing patients and families to feel more empowered and accepted. Support organizations, healthcare professionals, and patient advocates play a critical role in spreading knowledge and improving the visibility of blood disorders.

For example, initiatives that educate the public about **sickle cell disease** and its impact on patients can help reduce stigma and promote better understanding within communities. Advocating for policy changes to improve access to healthcare services, mental health resources, and financial assistance for those with chronic illnesses can also relieve some of the emotional and practical burdens associated with living with a blood disorder.

Conclusion

The emotional and psychological challenges of living with a blood disorder are undeniable. Anxiety, depression, and the emotional strain of managing a chronic illness can take a heavy toll on patients and their families. However, with proper support, coping strategies, and the right resources, patients can learn to manage the emotional impact of their conditions. **Psychological support, peer connections, self-care**, and **education** are vital tools in reducing mental health struggles and improving the quality of life for those affected by blood disorders.

As the healthcare community continues to prioritize the mental and emotional well-being of patients, the future of blood disorder treatment and care will be not only about physical healing but also about nurturing the emotional resilience needed to live well with chronic illness.

Chapter 35

The Family Impact: Genetic Disorders and Decision-Making

When a family is faced with a diagnosis of a hereditary blood disorder, the implications extend far beyond the individual patient. **Genetic blood disorders**, such as **sickle cell disease, thalassemia, hemophilia**, and **hemoglobinopathies**, not only affect the person diagnosed but can also deeply influence family dynamics, roles, and decision-making processes. These disorders, which are often passed down from one generation to the next, require families to confront difficult decisions, navigate complex emotional terrain, and consider long-term implications for their loved ones. This chapter explores the **family impact** of hereditary blood disorders and the multifaceted role of decision-making within families coping with these conditions.

The Emotional Weight of Hereditary Diagnosis

A diagnosis of a genetic blood disorder can create a ripple effect through a family. In many cases, these conditions are inherited in an **autosomal recessive** or **X-linked** pattern, meaning that both parents are usually carriers of the defective gene, even if they are asymptomatic. When a child is diagnosed with a hereditary blood disorder, parents may feel an overwhelming sense of **guilt, shock,** and **responsibility**. The emotional weight is especially heavy when one or both parents feel they could have prevented the condition through earlier knowledge, testing, or making different choices.

For example, **thalassemia**, which is most common in people of Mediterranean, Middle Eastern, and Southeast Asian descent, may be a condition that parents are unaware of before having children. When one or both parents are carriers of the thalassemia trait, the risk of passing on the disease to their child increases. A diagnosis of **thalassemia major**, which requires regular blood transfusions, iron chelation therapy, and lifelong management, can be devastating not only to the child but also to the parents, who are left grappling with the reality of the child's future and the medical needs they will face throughout their lives.

Similarly, families affected by **sickle cell disease**, which is inherited in an autosomal recessive pattern, are often affected by the same emotional turmoil. The parents' worry about their child experiencing painful crises, organ damage, and potential shortened life expectancy can be compounded by a sense of helplessness and despair. These emotions can lead to **stress, anxiety,** and **depression** within the family unit. The knowledge that the condition will likely affect future generations, creating an ongoing cycle of challenges, can create a sense of helplessness that feels difficult to overcome.

Decision-Making in the Context of Genetic Disorders

Decision-making in families with a hereditary blood disorder is multifaceted and often fraught with complexity. From prenatal testing to choices about medical care, the decisions that families make can be overwhelming. The presence of a **genetic blood disorder** adds an additional layer of uncertainty and difficulty to these decisions.

One of the first decisions many families face is whether or not to undergo **genetic counseling** or **genetic testing**. When parents are carriers of a genetic blood disorder, they may face the choice of whether to have **prenatal screening** or **preimplantation genetic diagnosis (PGD)** during pregnancy. These options allow parents to determine if their child will inherit the condition before birth. While some families opt for prenatal testing to prepare for the challenges ahead, others may struggle with the potential ethical and emotional consequences of knowing about a diagnosis before birth. The decision of whether to proceed with testing can strain family relationships, as opinions may differ on how much information is too much and whether knowing early will impact the choices made later on.

In cases where a child is already diagnosed with a hereditary blood disorder, decisions surrounding **medical care** and **treatment plans** are of paramount importance. Blood disorders such as **hemophilia** require families to make critical decisions about how to manage bleeding episodes, whether to use clotting factor treatments, and how to balance risk and safety. Families must also make decisions about the child's lifestyle, activities, and what precautions should be in place to prevent bleeding or injury. These decisions, while focused on the child's immediate needs, also affect the broader family dynamic as parents may need to make lifestyle changes or sacrifices to ensure their child's health and well-being.

Impacts on Siblings and Extended Family

When a hereditary blood disorder affects a child, the entire family is affected—not just the parents. **Siblings** of the affected child often experience their own unique set of emotions. Siblings may feel **jealous, neglected**, or **resentful**, as the parents' attention is often focused on the child with the chronic health condition. For example, in families where a child is frequently hospitalized or requires continuous medical care, siblings may feel that their needs are overlooked. They may also worry about their own potential to inherit the condition, especially in cases of conditions like sickle cell disease, where the genetic risk is high.

While these feelings are normal, the emotional toll on siblings can lead to **social withdrawal, low self-esteem**, and even **behavioral problems**. Parents may find it difficult to balance the emotional needs of all their children, particularly when one child requires more attention due to their condition. Open communication, emotional support, and family counseling can help address these feelings and ensure that siblings feel valued and understood. It is also important for families to make intentional efforts to involve siblings in the care process, fostering a sense of teamwork and shared responsibility for the affected child's well-being.

The extended family, including **grandparents, aunts, uncles**, and **cousins**, may also experience emotional challenges when a hereditary blood disorder is present. These family members may struggle with their own feelings of guilt or responsibility, especially if they are carriers of the condition and have passed it down through generations. Extended family members often want to help but may feel uncertain about how to do so. In some cases, grandparents may feel helpless in offering support, unsure of how to contribute to the child's care or the family's emotional needs. Encouraging open communication and educating extended family members about the disorder can help foster understanding and provide them with the tools they need to support the family.

Ethical and Moral Considerations

Hereditary blood disorders also introduce ethical and moral dilemmas into the decision-making process. Some families may wrestle with the decision to **conceive another child** after one child has been diagnosed with a genetic condition. In some cases, parents may decide to undergo **genetic testing** to determine the chances of having another child with the same disorder. Some families may choose to pursue **genetic selection** or **preimplantation genetic diagnosis (PGD)** to select embryos that do not carry the genetic mutation. While these decisions can provide families with a sense of control and the possibility of avoiding the challenges of raising a child with a hereditary blood disorder, they can also be ethically controversial and lead to intense moral debates.

For families dealing with conditions like **sickle cell disease**, which can have a severe impact on a person's quality of life, the decision about whether to have more children may be influenced by the experiences of the firstborn. Some parents may feel compelled to have more children, hoping for a **healthy sibling** who might serve as a **stem cell donor** or offer other forms of support to the affected child. While this decision is often made with the best of intentions, it raises complex ethical questions about **family planning** and the motivations behind conception.

Additionally, **bone marrow transplants** or **stem cell therapies** may offer potential cures for some genetic blood disorders, but they are not without risks. The decision to pursue these treatments is often weighed heavily by families, as the procedure can be invasive and have long-term consequences. Deciding whether to proceed with such treatments involves a careful assessment of the risks, benefits, and potential outcomes, both for the affected child and the family as a whole.

Support Systems for Families

Families dealing with hereditary blood disorders benefit from comprehensive support systems that help them navigate the emotional, social, and medical challenges they face. **Genetic counseling** plays an essential role in helping families understand the genetic basis of the condition and the potential risks to future generations. Genetic counselors provide valuable information about inheritance patterns, the likelihood of recurrence, and the available options for family planning. They also help families process the emotional aspects of having a child with a hereditary condition and prepare them for the practical realities of managing the condition.

In addition to medical and genetic counseling, **family therapy** can be an essential tool for addressing the emotional and relational aspects of living with a hereditary blood disorder. Therapy provides a safe space for family members to express their feelings, address interpersonal conflicts, and strengthen communication. Families who engage in therapy are often better equipped to handle the stresses of caregiving, sibling rivalry, and decision-making related to the child's condition.

Support groups, both online and in-person, offer a sense of solidarity and shared experience. Connecting with other families facing similar challenges can provide emotional relief, as families realize they are not alone in their struggles. Support groups offer the opportunity to share advice, resources, and coping strategies, and to find comfort in knowing that others have walked the same path.

Conclusion

Hereditary blood disorders have a profound impact not only on the individual patient but also on the entire family. The emotional toll of diagnosis, the weight of decision-making, and the challenges of coping with a lifelong condition can strain family dynamics, cause feelings of guilt, and affect the roles and relationships within the family. However, with the right resources, open communication, and strong support systems, families can navigate the complexities of hereditary blood disorders together. By making informed decisions, seeking counseling, and engaging with others who share their experiences, families can find strength in unity and resilience, ensuring that they face the future with hope, understanding, and love.

Chapter 36

Building Support Systems for Blood Disorder Patients

Living with a blood disorder is often a journey marked by medical appointments, treatments, emotional challenges, and physical hurdles. Whether dealing with conditions like **sickle cell anemia**, **hemophilia**, **thalassemia**, **anemia**, or **leukemia**, individuals and families can often feel isolated or overwhelmed by the daily demands of managing these conditions. One of the most important aspects of successfully managing a blood disorder is establishing strong, multifaceted **support systems**. These networks help patients navigate their challenges, improve their emotional well-being, and foster a sense of community and hope. This chapter explores the significance of building support systems for blood disorder patients, discussing the various types of support, how to cultivate them, and the transformative power of strong, supportive relationships.

The Need for Support Systems

When an individual is diagnosed with a blood disorder, it affects not only their physical health but also their emotional and social well-being. Patients often face a range of psychological challenges, including feelings of **isolation**, **anxiety**, **depression**, and **fear**. The unpredictability of blood disorders, particularly those with acute symptoms like **sickle cell crises** or **bleeding episodes** in hemophilia, can cause constant worry about the future. The long-term nature of many blood disorders also means that individuals must continuously manage their health, which can be physically and emotionally exhausting.

Without proper emotional and practical support, these challenges can become overwhelming. That is why building robust support systems is crucial. A support system for someone living with a blood disorder provides both **practical assistance** and **emotional comfort**, helping patients to feel empowered, understood, and less alone in their journey. It is important to recognize that support systems need to be diverse, encompassing different types of support to meet the varied needs of patients.

The Types of Support for Blood Disorder Patients

Emotional support forms the foundation of a strong support system. It involves providing understanding, empathy, and a listening ear. Family members, friends, and support groups play a crucial role in offering emotional reassurance during difficult times. Patients benefit from knowing that they have people who are genuinely concerned about their well-being and who understand their unique struggles. Emotional support fosters resilience and provides patients with the mental strength they need to manage their condition day-to-day.

For individuals living with chronic blood disorders, such as **thalassemia** or **hemophilia**, the emotional toll can be significant. Families and loved ones must actively engage in **open communication**, allowing patients to share their fears, frustrations, and hopes without judgment. Just as important is the ability of family members to listen without trying to "fix" everything—sometimes, patients simply need a compassionate presence to help them feel heard and validated.

In some cases, professional counseling or therapy can be incredibly beneficial. **Psychologists** or **therapists** who specialize in chronic illness can help patients work through feelings of **grief, loss, anger**, or **trauma** related to living with a blood disorder. They can also teach coping mechanisms to manage the psychological challenges associated with living with a long-term illness.

Practical Support:
Managing a blood disorder often requires numerous medical treatments, including regular visits to healthcare providers, blood transfusions, medication administration, and at-home care. For many patients, especially those with complex or severe conditions, these tasks can become overwhelming. **Practical support** involves the hands-on assistance needed to manage these activities effectively.

Support can come from various sources. Family members and friends can step in to help with transportation to medical appointments, assist with preparing medications, or provide childcare during hospital stays. In cases where the patient is too ill to attend school or work, support from loved ones can also help with daily tasks like cooking, cleaning, and running errands. For patients who experience severe symptoms, having reliable help is essential to ensure they can continue living with some degree of normalcy.

For patients with conditions such as **sickle cell disease,** where **pain crises** can come on unexpectedly and require immediate medical intervention, knowing that someone is there to help in an emergency situation can be invaluable. Practical support also extends to people who can help organize and track the patient's medical history, test results, and appointments, making it easier to coordinate care with healthcare providers.

Social Support:

The role of social connections in managing a blood disorder cannot be overstated. **Social support** involves the relationships patients maintain with others outside of their immediate family and healthcare team, such as friends, colleagues, and peers. Social networks can provide a sense of belonging and acceptance, which is vital for emotional well-being.

For patients with chronic illnesses, social support also means connecting with others who truly understand their experiences. **Support groups** are often an ideal place to find like-minded individuals who are facing similar challenges. In these groups, patients can share advice, exchange coping strategies, and celebrate each other's victories. Peer support can also be a source of hope, especially for individuals newly diagnosed with a blood disorder who may be struggling to understand their future prospects.

There are several types of support groups available, from those organized by disease-specific organizations to online communities. The anonymity and accessibility of online platforms allow people from all over the world to connect with others who understand their journey, offering support that transcends geographical boundaries.

In addition to formal support groups, having friends and a social network outside the realm of illness is essential. Social activities that are unrelated to the patient's health offer an opportunity for patients to experience **joy**, **distraction**, and **normalcy**. Encouraging patients to continue participating in hobbies, volunteer work, or community activities is vital for preserving a sense of identity and self-worth.

Medical Support:

In addition to emotional, practical, and social support, **medical support** is fundamental for individuals living with blood disorders. A well-coordinated healthcare team ensures that patients receive the most effective treatments and care. This team may consist of **hematologists**, **nurses**, **social workers**, and other specialists who have expertise in blood disorders.

Effective **patient-provider communication** is at the heart of strong medical support. Patients must feel that they are in partnership with their healthcare providers, that their voices are heard, and that they are involved in decisions regarding their treatment plans. A positive, trusting relationship with healthcare professionals can lead to improved treatment outcomes and a higher quality of life.

For patients with **sickle cell disease, hemophilia**, or **anemia**, treatment often involves a combination of medications, lifestyle changes, and, in some cases, blood transfusions. Having a dedicated medical team that understands the nuances of the patient's condition is crucial for providing the right care and intervention when needed.

Moreover, specialized **genetic counseling** can be an essential part of the medical support system for families with hereditary blood disorders. Genetic counselors provide guidance on understanding the genetic basis of a disease, the risks to future children, and the potential for targeted therapies, such as **gene therapy**, that may become available as treatment options.

The Role of Advocacy Organizations and Community Resources

Numerous advocacy organizations play a pivotal role in supporting individuals living with blood disorders. These organizations often provide a wealth of resources, including educational materials, financial assistance, and advocacy for better treatment options and healthcare access. Some well-known organizations, such as the **National Hemophilia Foundation**, the **Sickle Cell Disease Association of America**, and **Thalassemia International Federation**, offer extensive support for patients and families, connecting them with local chapters, online communities, and expert guidance.

Additionally, these organizations often help fund research efforts aimed at finding new treatments or cures for blood disorders, further empowering patients by allowing them to become active participants in advancing the field of blood disorder medicine.

Building Support Systems: A Collaborative Effort

Building a strong support system for blood disorder patients is not something that happens overnight. It is a continuous, collaborative effort involving patients, families, healthcare professionals, advocacy organizations, and communities. Families must work together to identify their needs, engage in open communication, and seek out the resources that will help them cope with the challenges of living with a chronic blood condition. Likewise, healthcare providers must actively listen to the unique concerns of their patients and collaborate to create a holistic, patient-centered care plan.

By prioritizing emotional, social, and practical support, patients with blood disorders can feel empowered and better equipped to manage the day-to-day realities of their condition. Families, peers, and professionals must create a network of support that is tailored to the individual patient's needs, offering assistance in ways that respect their dignity, autonomy, and goals for the future.

Conclusion

Support systems are the bedrock upon which patients living with blood disorders can build a healthier, more balanced life. By fostering **strong emotional connections**, ensuring **practical help** in managing the condition, and maintaining **social ties**, families and individuals can face the challenges of chronic illness with confidence, resilience, and hope. It is essential for all those involved in a blood disorder patient's life—family, friends, healthcare professionals, and advocacy groups—to work collaboratively to build a network of support that not only aids in managing the disorder but also enriches the overall quality of life. A robust support system transforms a difficult journey into one filled with strength, connection, and possibility.

Chapter 37

Advocacy and Awareness: Fighting for Better Treatment

Advocacy is the voice of change, and when it comes to blood disorders, it plays an essential role in improving treatment options, increasing awareness, and securing funding for crucial research. The complexity and diversity of blood disorders, ranging from genetic conditions like **sickle cell anemia** and **thalassemia** to acquired conditions such as **leukemia** and **hemophilia**, mean that individuals living with these disorders often face significant challenges. These challenges extend beyond the medical treatment itself to include a lack of awareness, insufficient funding for research, and gaps in healthcare policy that can hinder access to proper care.

This chapter explores the significance of **advocacy** in the realm of blood disorders, emphasizing how efforts to raise awareness, secure funding for research, and push for policy change can significantly improve the lives of those affected. By understanding the importance of advocacy, individuals, families, and organizations can be empowered to act as agents of change and help bring about tangible improvements in the diagnosis, treatment, and care of blood disorder patients.

The Role of Advocacy in Blood Disorder Awareness

Advocacy is crucial in shining a light on the often-overlooked issues faced by individuals with blood disorders. Many blood disorders are rare, complex, or misunderstood by the general public, which can lead to social stigma, misdiagnosis, delayed treatment, and a lack of understanding. For example, **sickle cell disease** primarily affects individuals of African, Mediterranean, Middle Eastern, and Indian ancestry, yet its symptoms are often mistaken for other, more common conditions. Similarly, **hemophilia** is commonly underdiagnosed, and the awareness about **von Willebrand disease** remains relatively low, despite being one of the most common inherited bleeding disorders.

Advocacy groups, both local and international, are pivotal in raising public awareness and educating communities about the symptoms, risks, and impacts of these diseases. **Awareness campaigns** that focus on highlighting the challenges faced by people with blood disorders help dispel myths, reduce stigma, and increase understanding. These campaigns often use social media, public service announcements, and educational materials to reach a wide audience and bring the issues into public discourse.

Through increased awareness, advocacy not only helps patients feel less isolated but also enables them to be recognized by healthcare providers, insurance companies, and policy-makers as individuals with distinct medical needs. Without the consistent efforts of advocacy groups, many patients would remain invisible in the broader healthcare system, making it even harder for them to access the treatments and services they need.

Research Funding: The Lifeblood of Advancements

In the realm of medical science, research is the driving force behind new and improved treatments. For individuals with blood disorders, research holds the key to finding cures, improving disease management strategies, and ultimately enhancing the quality of life. However, despite the immense importance of research in blood disorder treatment, **funding** remains a significant barrier.

Blood disorders, particularly rare ones, often receive less attention from both government and private funding sources compared to more common conditions like cancer or heart disease. Inadequate research funding leads to slower advancements in treatment options, less understanding of the underlying mechanisms of these diseases, and fewer breakthroughs in **genetic therapies** or **biologics**. It also hampers the development of **personalized medicine** approaches, which could significantly improve patient outcomes by tailoring treatments to individual genetic profiles.

Advocacy plays a pivotal role in securing funding for blood disorder research. Advocacy groups often collaborate with medical research institutions, healthcare providers, and government agencies to create awareness about the funding gap in blood disorder research. They may organize fundraising events, petition for increased government funding, or partner with pharmaceutical companies to accelerate the development of new therapies.

One notable example of successful advocacy is the push for **gene therapy** in the treatment of diseases like **sickle cell anemia** and **hemophilia**. Thanks to increased awareness and funding, **clinical trials** for gene therapy have advanced, offering hope for a future where some blood disorders may be cured at the genetic level. Advocacy has also been crucial in securing funding for **bone marrow**

transplant programs and **blood transfusion research**, which have saved countless lives.

Policy Changes: Shaping Healthcare for Blood Disorder Patients

Beyond raising awareness and securing funding for research, advocacy is instrumental in advocating for **policy changes** that directly affect the lives of people with blood disorders. Healthcare policy plays a critical role in determining access to medical services, treatments, and medications. In many parts of the world, people living with blood disorders often face difficulties in accessing the care they need, due to high treatment costs, limited healthcare infrastructure, and gaps in policy.

For example, in countries with fragmented healthcare systems, the cost of blood transfusions or **clotting factor replacement** therapy can be prohibitively expensive. Advocacy organizations work tirelessly to lobby for **policy reforms** that make healthcare more accessible to individuals with blood disorders. This includes pushing for greater insurance coverage, subsidies for life-saving treatments, and better access to medical specialists.

Another important area of policy advocacy is **access to genetic counseling** and **genetic testing**. As genetic research continues to advance, the ability to diagnose and manage blood disorders through genetic screening has become a crucial part of patient care. Advocacy for policies that ensure broad access to genetic testing and counseling is essential to ensuring that all individuals with blood disorders, regardless of income or location, can benefit from the latest diagnostic tools.

Furthermore, many advocacy groups are working to ensure that blood disorder treatments and healthcare services are recognized as priorities in national healthcare agendas. This can involve efforts to include blood disorder treatment in **national health insurance programs**, especially in low-resource settings where patients might otherwise go untreated.

Patient Advocacy: Empowering Individuals and Families

Patient advocacy is a critical component of the broader movement for better treatment of blood disorders. This form of advocacy empowers patients and their families to take an active role in their healthcare journey. Patient advocacy can involve supporting individuals in understanding their rights, navigating the healthcare system, and ensuring they have access to the best possible care.

Support groups and patient advocates work closely with families to help them understand their diagnosis, treatment options, and potential outcomes. In addition to offering emotional support, patient advocates help to connect families with healthcare providers, ensure that patients' voices are heard in their treatment plans, and guide them through the maze of healthcare policies, insurance procedures, and medical options.

Advocacy also extends beyond healthcare settings, as patients and their families often become powerful voices in the fight for policy changes and research funding. When blood disorder patients and their families share their personal stories, they help humanize the issues and create a deeper understanding of the day-to-day struggles of living with these conditions. These personal stories are a powerful tool in pushing for changes in both public perception and government policy.

The Global Advocacy Movement

While advocacy efforts at the national level are critical, blood disorder patients also benefit from global advocacy initiatives. The world is home to millions of individuals living with blood disorders, and global advocacy ensures that even the most marginalized patients have access to treatments and support. International organizations such as the **World Federation of Hemophilia**, **Sickle Cell Disease International**, and **Thalassemia International Federation** play a vital role in connecting advocacy groups across borders, enabling collaboration, and fostering a shared global mission to improve care for people with blood disorders.

Global advocacy efforts focus on harmonizing treatment protocols, ensuring access to blood products and medications, and advancing international research efforts. Through partnerships with organizations like the **World Health Organization (WHO)** and **global health initiatives**, advocacy groups can push for broader healthcare reforms that benefit blood disorder patients worldwide. These initiatives often focus on making treatments accessible in resource-limited settings, where patients may not have access to the most advanced therapies or even basic care.

Conclusion

Advocacy is a crucial tool in improving the lives of individuals living with blood disorders. From raising awareness about the challenges patients face to securing funding for vital research and pushing for policy changes that improve access to treatment, advocacy plays a central role in bringing about change. Patient advocates, families, healthcare providers, and global organizations must continue to work together to ensure that blood disorder patients receive the care they need, the research they deserve, and the public awareness they require. The fight for better treatment for blood disorder patients is not just about medical progress; it's about empowering individuals and families to live healthier, more fulfilling lives despite the challenges they face. The future of blood disorder care lies in the collective efforts of advocates who work tirelessly to drive positive change, one step at a time.

Chapter 38

A Day in the Life: Personal Stories of Blood Disorder Patients

Living with a blood disorder is an experience that shapes every aspect of daily life, from physical health to emotional well-being and social interactions. For many individuals, managing these conditions requires more than just medical treatment; it involves navigating a world where the challenges of the disorder often go unseen by others. Each patient's journey is unique, and their stories provide powerful insights into the realities of living with conditions such as **anemia, sickle cell disease, hemophilia,** and **thrombosis.**

In this chapter, we will hear from individuals with these disorders, each of whom will share their personal experiences, challenges, and the resilience they demonstrate every day. These stories, drawn from diverse perspectives, illuminate the complexities of living with blood disorders and provide inspiration for others facing similar battles.

Maria's Story: Living with Iron-Deficiency Anemia

Maria, a 34-year-old teacher from Texas, had always been an active person, balancing her busy career and home life with ease. However, in her early 30s, she began to notice unusual fatigue. She chalked it up to the stresses of her job, but as the months passed, the exhaustion became overwhelming. She found it harder to keep up with her students, and even simple tasks like grocery shopping left her feeling drained.

"I remember walking up the stairs one day and realizing I couldn't catch my breath. I felt weak all over," Maria recalls. "I went to my doctor, and after several blood tests, I was diagnosed with iron-deficiency anemia."

Iron-deficiency anemia is one of the most common types of anemia, caused by a lack of iron in the body, leading to insufficient red blood cells to carry oxygen throughout the body. For Maria, the diagnosis was both a relief and a challenge. While it explained her fatigue and shortness of breath, it also meant she would need to make significant changes to her lifestyle.

Maria's treatment plan included iron supplements, a diet rich in iron, and addressing underlying issues like menstrual irregularities, which had been contributing to her condition. "I had to re-evaluate my eating habits and make sure I was getting enough nutrients," she says. "Iron-rich foods like spinach, lentils, and red meat became a staple in my diet."

While her symptoms have improved with treatment, Maria has learned that managing her anemia requires ongoing vigilance. "I have to be proactive about my health now. If I feel tired or weak, I know I need to check my iron levels. It's all about listening to my body and not ignoring the signs."

James's Journey: A Life with Sickle Cell Disease

For James, a 28-year-old graphic designer from Atlanta, living with **sickle cell disease** is a lifelong struggle. Sickle cell anemia is a genetic disorder in which the red blood cells become rigid and shaped like a crescent moon, leading to painful blockages in blood vessels and reduced oxygen flow to organs. The pain crises that result can be excruciating and unpredictable, often leading to hospitalizations.

"I was diagnosed with sickle cell when I was a baby, but I didn't fully understand what it meant until I was older," James says. "As a kid, I would miss school often because of the pain. It was frustrating. I wanted to play sports and be active like my friends, but I couldn't."

As James entered adulthood, the pain crises continued, and he learned to manage them by staying hydrated, avoiding extreme temperatures, and taking prescribed medications. Despite these precautions, he often faces flare-ups that disrupt his life. "I know when a pain crisis is coming because my body starts to feel heavy, like everything is weighed down," he shares. "It's a deep ache that won't go away, and the only thing I can do is go to the hospital for pain management."

Although sickle cell disease requires regular monitoring and the possibility of complications such as stroke or organ damage, James has managed to build a fulfilling life. He remains active in his community, advocating for better access to care and increased research funding for sickle cell. "It's not easy, but I've learned to adapt and keep pushing forward. I want to help others with sickle cell disease know they're not alone."

Eva's Experience: Hemophilia and the Fear of Bleeding

Eva, a 42-year-old mother of two from New York, has **hemophilia**, a rare bleeding disorder that prevents blood from clotting properly. For Eva, this means that even a minor injury can lead to excessive bleeding, bruising, or internal bleeding. Throughout her life, she has faced challenges in managing this condition, often worrying about everyday activities that others take for granted.

"I was diagnosed with hemophilia when I was a baby, but it wasn't until I was a toddler that my parents began to realize something was wrong. I would bleed for longer than usual after minor cuts or bruises," Eva explains.

Managing hemophilia has meant a lifelong regimen of **clotting factor infusions** to help her blood clot properly. These treatments, which must be administered regularly, have become a routine part of her life. "It's a balancing act," she says. "On one hand, I need the infusions to prevent bleeding episodes, but on the other, I have to be careful not to overdo it physically, as even a small injury can turn into something serious."

As an adult, Eva has adapted her lifestyle by learning to manage risks, such as avoiding contact sports and taking extra precautions when traveling or engaging in physical activities. "I have to think ahead," she says. "Before I go on a trip, I make sure I have all my supplies, including my infusions, and I avoid activities that could put me at risk for injuries."

For Eva, the emotional toll of hemophilia can be as challenging as the physical limitations. "There are times when I feel anxious about bleeding or injuring myself. I worry about my kids and the example I'm setting for them. But I also want them to understand that despite my condition, I can still live a full life."

Lucas's Struggle: Deep Vein Thrombosis and Pulmonary Embolism

Lucas, a 55-year-old construction manager from Chicago, was diagnosed with **deep vein thrombosis (DVT)** after experiencing severe pain and swelling in his left leg. DVT occurs when a blood clot forms in a deep vein, typically in the leg, and can lead to serious complications like **pulmonary embolism (PE)** if the clot travels to the lungs. For Lucas, the diagnosis was a wake-up call that forced him to make significant lifestyle changes.

"I had no idea what DVT was until it happened to me," Lucas shares. "One day, my leg started swelling up, and it was really painful. I thought I had just pulled a muscle, but when it didn't get better, I went to the hospital and found out I had a blood clot."

Lucas was immediately treated with anticoagulants to prevent the clot from traveling to his lungs and causing a pulmonary embolism, a potentially fatal condition. In addition to the medication, he was advised to make changes to his daily habits, including **increasing physical activity**, **losing weight**, and avoiding prolonged periods of immobility. "I used to sit for hours on end, especially when I was working on paperwork," he says. "Now, I make it a point to get up and walk around every hour, and I've started swimming to improve circulation."

Lucas's experience with DVT has had a lasting impact on his outlook on health. "I've learned the hard way that we can't take our bodies for granted. I make sure to take care of myself now, and I keep a close eye on my health."

Conclusion: Resilience and Hope

The stories shared in this chapter reveal the diverse challenges faced by individuals with blood disorders. Each person's experience is unique, but there are common threads of resilience, determination, and hope that run through them. Despite the physical, emotional, and social hurdles they face, these individuals continue to fight for their health, advocate for better treatment, and lead meaningful lives.

Living with a blood disorder is not easy, but it's clear from these personal stories that people are not defined by their condition. They adapt, persevere, and find ways to thrive despite the daily challenges. By sharing these stories, we gain a deeper understanding of the courage and strength required to live with a blood disorder, and we are reminded that, through advocacy, awareness, and ongoing research, progress is being made toward better treatments and improved quality of life for all those affected.

Chapter 39

Overcoming the Stigma: Living with a Visible or Invisible Illness

Living with a blood disorder can be challenging in ways that go beyond the physical symptoms and medical treatment. For many individuals, the emotional and psychological toll of dealing with stigma, misconceptions, and a lack of understanding about their condition can be just as debilitating as the disease itself. Whether the condition is **visible**, such as the frequent bruising or joint swelling in individuals with **hemophilia**, or **invisible**, like the fatigue and pain experienced by those with **sickle cell disease** or **anemia**, the stigma surrounding these disorders can significantly impact a person's quality of life.

This chapter delves into the realities of living with a blood disorder in a world that often lacks awareness and empathy. We will explore the social and emotional challenges these individuals face, how they navigate prejudice, and what they are doing to foster understanding, acceptance, and support for themselves and others living with similar conditions.

The Silent Struggles of Invisible Illnesses

One of the most common struggles for individuals with blood disorders is that many of these conditions are invisible. **Sickle cell disease**, **iron-deficiency anemia**, **thrombophilia**, and **chronic hemophilia** may not present any obvious outward signs, especially during periods of remission or when treatment is effective. To an outsider, a person with an invisible illness might appear perfectly healthy, leading to a dangerous misconception that they are not truly sick or that they are exaggerating their symptoms.

Sickle cell disease is a prime example of an invisible illness. Individuals with this genetic blood disorder suffer from **painful sickle cell crises**, but there is no visible indicator that they are experiencing this severe discomfort. For many, the lack of visible symptoms can lead to frustration when others downplay their struggles or misunderstand their pain.

"I've had people tell me I look fine, so they assume I'm not really in pain," says Malik, a 26-year-old with sickle cell disease. "I get it all the time—'You look great!' or 'But you don't look sick.' What they don't understand is that the pain is internal, and I could be having a crisis without anyone even knowing. That misunderstanding can make me feel isolated and misunderstood."

The **stigma of invisibility** can lead to feelings of isolation, shame, and frustration. It can also discourage people from seeking support or explaining their condition to others. Some may even avoid discussing their illness out of fear of being dismissed or not taken seriously.

"For me, the hardest part was explaining why I had to leave work early or miss social events," says Sarah, a 34-year-old woman with **iron-deficiency anemia**. "People would often brush it off and tell me to eat more iron-rich foods, as if that's all it took to fix it. It's not that simple, and that lack of understanding can make you feel like you're not being heard."

Visible Blood Disorders: Misconceptions and Judgment

On the other hand, individuals with **visible blood disorders** face a different set of challenges. **Hemophilia**, for example, is a disorder that prevents blood from clotting properly, leading to frequent bruising and bleeding episodes. The visible signs of the disease—bruises, joint swelling, or bandages—can often prompt unwelcome questions or judgments.

"I've had people ask me, 'What happened to you? Did you fall?' or 'Why are you always getting bruises?' They don't understand that it's not because I'm clumsy, it's because my blood doesn't clot properly," shares Thomas, a 42-year-old living with **hemophilia**. "The assumptions that people make can be frustrating, especially when they don't take the time to ask or learn about what I have. It often feels like they see the bruises first, and not the person."

In addition to the assumptions made based on visible symptoms, people with visible blood disorders may face embarrassment or self-consciousness. The frequent need for medical interventions, such as injections or treatments for swelling, may draw unwanted attention and further intensify the stigma.

The Fear of Being Defined by the Disorder

For many individuals with blood disorders, the fear of being defined by their condition can lead to an emotional struggle between seeking support and wanting to maintain a sense of independence and normalcy. Living with a chronic illness—whether visible or invisible—can be emotionally taxing, and individuals may feel the need to constantly explain themselves to friends, family, colleagues, and even strangers.

"I don't want people to think that hemophilia defines me," says Anita, a 30-year-old professional with hemophilia. "It's something I have, but it's not all that I am. But sometimes it feels like people only see me as 'the girl with the bleeding disorder' and not as a person with hopes, dreams, and a career."

This fear of being reduced to a diagnosis can be especially challenging in the workplace, where discrimination, lack of accommodations, and even subtle biases can arise. "It's difficult in meetings when I have to sit down and rest for a while, or when I need to take a break because I'm in pain," says Malik. "People don't always understand, and I've been passed over for promotions because of it. They just don't know how to accommodate my needs."

The challenge of feeling **"othered"** or separated from others because of one's illness is a constant emotional burden. However, as more people speak out about their experiences, the hope is that society will become more compassionate and aware of the complexities of living with a blood disorder.

Breaking the Silence: Advocacy and Education

While stigma and misconceptions are prevalent, there is also a growing movement of individuals and organizations advocating for change. **Advocacy** is key to breaking down the barriers of misunderstanding and stigma that surround blood disorders, and many patients are taking matters into their own hands.

Non-profit organizations dedicated to raising awareness about blood disorders, such as the **Sickle Cell Disease Association of America** and the **National Hemophilia Foundation**, are doing critical work to educate the public, provide resources for patients, and fight for policy changes to improve access to care and research funding. These organizations also serve as a vital support network for people living with blood disorders.

Moreover, social media has become a powerful tool for patients to share their stories, connect with others, and raise awareness. Many individuals use platforms like Instagram, Facebook, and Twitter to document their journey with blood disorders, offering a glimpse into their lives and providing a sense of solidarity for others facing similar challenges.

"Social media has been a game-changer for me," says Sarah. "Through my posts about living with anemia, I've connected with so many people who understand what I'm going through. It's empowering to know I'm not alone and that I can help others feel heard."

The Importance of Compassionate Support

Another powerful way to combat stigma is through compassion and open communication. For patients with blood disorders, having a strong support system—whether it's friends, family, or healthcare providers—is essential. Feeling understood and accepted can significantly improve mental health and quality of life.

"I've learned to be more open about my condition with my family and friends," says Eva, a 38-year-old mother living with hemophilia. "When they understand what I go through, they're more supportive. I don't have to explain myself all the time, and it's one less thing I have to worry about. That sense of support really helps with the emotional strain."

Empathy and awareness in the workplace, schools, and community can go a long way in reducing stigma. For example, employers who understand the needs of employees with blood disorders can provide accommodations such as flexible work hours or medical leave. Teachers who are educated about the signs and symptoms of blood disorders can create a supportive environment for students.

Finding Empowerment and Hope

While stigma and misunderstanding remain challenges for many living with blood disorders, countless individuals are learning to rise above them. By embracing their identity as more than just their illness, patients are taking control of their narrative and finding ways to live fulfilling, empowered lives.

Ultimately, the key to overcoming the stigma surrounding blood disorders lies in education, empathy, and open dialogue. As awareness grows, more people will understand that blood disorders do not define a person's worth, and that those living with these conditions are deserving of respect, support, and the same opportunities as anyone else.

For individuals with blood disorders, each day is a testament to their strength and resilience. They are breaking down barriers, challenging misconceptions, and showing the world that they are not their diagnosis—they are individuals with unique stories, dreams, and contributions to make.

In the words of Anita, "It's a journey. And every day, I'm fighting to make it my own."

Chapter 40

The Role of Artificial Blood

The pursuit of **artificial blood** is one of the most fascinating and potentially transformative areas of medical research. It promises to not only revolutionize how we treat blood disorders but also offer groundbreaking solutions to a problem that has plagued the global healthcare system for decades: the chronic shortage of donated blood. Blood transfusions have been a cornerstone of medicine for over a century, helping to save countless lives in emergencies, surgeries, and treatments for blood-related conditions. Yet despite its life-saving role, the availability of blood for transfusion remains a significant challenge. The hope is that artificial blood could bridge this gap, creating a safe, efficient, and accessible alternative to human blood that can be used in medical settings across the world.

In this chapter, we will explore the concept of artificial blood, the science behind its development, the hurdles that must be overcome, and the potential it holds for the future of blood disorder treatment and healthcare in general.

Understanding Artificial Blood: What It Is and How It Works

Artificial blood, also known as **blood substitutes**, refers to man-made products that mimic some of the functions of human blood. The two primary functions of blood that researchers aim to replicate in artificial blood are **oxygen transport** and **carbon dioxide removal**. These functions are crucial for sustaining life, and artificial blood is being designed to carry out these roles without the need for red blood cells, platelets, or plasma—components typically found in human blood.

There are two main categories of artificial blood under development:

1. **Hemoglobin-based oxygen carriers (HBOCs):** These synthetic blood products are designed to use hemoglobin, the oxygen-carrying protein in red blood cells, to transport oxygen throughout the body. Researchers have worked to develop purified hemoglobin derived from human or animal sources, and more recently, synthetic hemoglobin, to function as an oxygen carrier in the bloodstream. The goal is to create a product that can transport oxygen as effectively as red blood cells.

2. **Perfluorocarbons (PFCs):** Unlike HBOCs, perfluorocarbons do not rely on hemoglobin to transport oxygen. Instead, they dissolve oxygen and carbon dioxide, allowing for the direct exchange of gases. PFCs are synthetic molecules that can carry high volumes of oxygen, even in environments where hemoglobin may not be as effective, such as in low-oxygen conditions. One of the key advantages of PFCs is that they can be stored for long periods, even at room temperature, which could greatly enhance their usability in emergency settings.

Both of these products are designed to serve as **temporary substitutes** for human blood in situations where a transfusion is needed. They can be used in trauma cases, surgeries, and emergency medicine where blood loss is significant, or when a patient has a blood disorder that requires frequent transfusions. However, both types of artificial blood come with unique challenges in terms of efficacy, safety, and widespread use.

The Need for Artificial Blood

The **global blood shortage crisis** has been an ongoing issue for decades. Despite efforts to increase blood donations, the demand for blood outpaces the supply, particularly in developing nations. Blood is a perishable commodity, with a shelf life of only 35 to 42 days for red blood cells, making it difficult to ensure that hospitals always have the necessary supply on hand.

Moreover, blood donations are subject to seasonal fluctuations and rely on voluntary donations, which can be affected by factors such as donor availability, public awareness, and natural disasters. Additionally, some patients, such as those with **sickle cell disease**, **thalassemia**, or **hemophilia**, require frequent blood transfusions, which can further strain available supplies. For these individuals, access to regular blood transfusions is essential for managing their condition, yet the unpredictability of blood availability creates an ongoing challenge for healthcare providers and patients alike.

Artificial blood offers a potential solution to this problem by providing a **ready-made** and **easily accessible** alternative to human blood. Since artificial blood products could be stored for extended periods and potentially in more flexible conditions, they would be available when needed, without concerns about expiration dates or donor availability. This could prove particularly useful in emergency situations, military settings, and disaster relief operations, where rapid access to blood is critical to saving lives.

The Promise of Artificial Blood for Blood Disorder Patients

For individuals living with **blood disorders** like **sickle cell disease** and **thalassemia**, artificial blood has the potential to change the way their conditions are managed. Both of these conditions involve problems with red blood cells—whether it be sickle-shaped cells in sickle cell disease or defective hemoglobin in thalassemia—that can lead to painful episodes, organ damage, and other complications. Frequent blood transfusions are often necessary to manage these conditions, but they come with their own set of challenges, including the risk of **iron overload** (due to repeated transfusions) and complications from blood group incompatibility.

Artificial blood could serve as a **temporary alternative** to donor blood, providing patients with relief from the complications associated with frequent transfusions. For example, patients with **sickle cell disease** often require blood transfusions to manage **sickle cell crises** and reduce the risk of stroke or organ damage. However, receiving too many blood transfusions over time can lead to an accumulation of iron in the body, which can cause **organ toxicity**. By providing a synthetic blood substitute that could carry oxygen without the same risk of iron overload, artificial blood could help mitigate these risks.

For patients with **thalassemia**, who require lifelong blood transfusions to maintain normal levels of red blood cells, artificial blood could offer a more convenient and accessible treatment option. Since thalassemia patients often experience complications from both the disease and blood transfusions, having access to a safe and efficient synthetic blood product could significantly improve their quality of life and reduce the burden of frequent hospital visits.

Challenges in Developing Artificial Blood

Despite its potential, the development of artificial blood products has faced numerous challenges. The complexity of human blood and its myriad functions makes it difficult to replicate in a synthetic form. For example, human blood is not just responsible for oxygen transport; it also plays vital roles in immune defense, clotting, and maintaining the body's **acid-base balance**. Achieving a product that mimics these functions without the risks associated with donor blood has proven to be a monumental task.

Safety concerns are also a major hurdle. When developing artificial blood products, scientists must ensure that these substances do not trigger **immune**

reactions, which could result in dangerous side effects. Additionally, both hemoglobin-based carriers and perfluorocarbons can have side effects on the cardiovascular system, such as increasing blood pressure or causing vascular damage, which means they must be rigorously tested and refined before they can be widely used.

Another issue is **cost**. The process of creating synthetic blood is expensive, particularly when it involves the use of advanced technologies and engineering. Researchers must also consider the economic implications of mass production, ensuring that artificial blood can be affordable and accessible in low-resource settings, where the need for blood substitutes may be greatest.

Despite these challenges, researchers remain optimistic. Over the past few decades, there have been several breakthroughs in the development of artificial blood, with some products already undergoing clinical trials. Although these products are not yet ready for widespread use, the **future of artificial blood** looks promising, especially as technology continues to advance.

The Future of Artificial Blood

The potential impact of artificial blood on the treatment of **blood disorders** and healthcare as a whole is immense. Researchers believe that the future of blood substitutes lies in **personalized medicine**, where synthetic blood products could be designed to better match individual patients' needs. For example, a person with a rare blood type or a specific medical condition could receive artificial blood that is customized to meet their unique requirements. This could reduce the risks of complications associated with blood transfusions, such as **infections** or **reactions to incompatible blood types**.

In addition to **genetic engineering**, new **nanotechnology** and **bioprinting** techniques could further enhance the development of artificial blood. These technologies could allow for the creation of more advanced, efficient, and safer blood substitutes that could be tailored for specific diseases or treatments. For example, researchers are looking into the possibility of creating **biocompatible nanomaterials** that could mimic the structure and function of blood cells more precisely, opening new avenues for treating blood disorders with minimal risk.

As researchers continue to refine these technologies, artificial blood may one day become a routine component of **emergency care, blood disorder treatment**, and **trauma medicine**. In combination with other medical advances, artificial blood could help address the global blood shortage, offering a solution that saves lives, improves health outcomes, and reduces the burden on the healthcare system.

Conclusion

The development of artificial blood has the potential to change the face of modern medicine. While challenges remain, the future of synthetic blood holds great promise for treating individuals with blood disorders and solving the critical issue of blood shortages worldwide. For patients who rely on frequent transfusions to manage their conditions, artificial blood offers hope for a safer, more accessible treatment option. As research continues and the technology matures, the world may soon see the realization of this long-held medical dream: a reliable, sustainable alternative to human blood that can save lives and improve the quality of care for patients around the globe.

Chapter 41

Gene Therapy: A Breakthrough in Blood Disorder Treatment

In recent years, **gene therapy** has emerged as a groundbreaking medical advancement, offering new hope to patients suffering from inherited blood disorders. This revolutionary approach holds the potential to correct genetic mutations at the source, offering patients the possibility of a **cure** rather than just lifelong management of their condition. For disorders like **sickle cell disease**, **thalassemia**, and other genetic blood disorders, gene therapy could dramatically alter the way we approach treatment, moving from symptom management to potentially eliminating the root cause of these diseases.

In this chapter, we will explore the role of gene therapy in the treatment of blood disorders, examine how this innovative technology works, discuss its potential benefits and challenges, and consider what the future holds for patients with genetic blood disorders.

Understanding Gene Therapy: The Basics

At its core, gene therapy is a medical technique that involves modifying the **genetic material** within a person's cells to treat or prevent disease. The goal is to address the underlying cause of a disease by altering the **genes** that are defective or missing. In the case of **blood disorders**, this typically means either repairing or replacing the faulty genes responsible for producing abnormal blood cells or proteins.

Gene therapy can be applied in different ways depending on the condition being treated. In **in vivo** gene therapy, the therapy is delivered directly into the patient's body, where it targets specific cells or tissues. In **ex vivo** gene therapy, a patient's own cells are removed from the body, modified in a lab, and then reintroduced to the patient.

The most common method used in gene therapy for blood disorders is **gene editing**. This process involves using specialized tools, such as **CRISPR-Cas9**, to precisely alter specific genes in the patient's DNA. By editing these genes, scientists aim to correct genetic mutations that cause blood disorders, restoring normal blood cell production and function.

Gene Therapy for Sickle Cell Disease: A Promising Cure

Sickle cell disease (SCD) is one of the most well-known and devastating **genetic blood disorders**. It is caused by a mutation in the **hemoglobin gene** that leads to the production of **sickle-shaped red blood cells**, which can block blood flow, cause severe pain, and lead to a variety of life-threatening complications. For decades, treatment for sickle cell disease has primarily focused on **pain management, blood transfusions**, and **preventing complications**. Bone marrow transplants are the only potential cure for the disease, but they come with risks, including finding a compatible donor, and are not available for all patients.

In recent years, gene therapy has shown great promise as a potential cure for sickle cell disease. Researchers have focused on two main strategies:

1. **Correcting the Sickle Cell Mutation:** The first approach involves directly correcting the mutation in the patient's **hemoglobin gene**. In this method, doctors use gene editing tools, such as CRISPR, to **edit the sickle cell mutation** and replace it with a healthy version of the gene. This process allows the patient's body to produce normal, round red blood cells, eliminating the symptoms of sickle cell disease.
2. **Reactivating Fetal Hemoglobin Production:** The second approach aims to induce the production of **fetal hemoglobin**, a type of hemoglobin that is normally produced during fetal development but is largely absent in adults. By introducing a gene that reactivates the production of fetal hemoglobin, researchers hope to compensate for the defective adult hemoglobin that causes the sickle-shaped cells. Fetal hemoglobin has a much lower tendency to sickle, and increasing its levels in patients with sickle cell disease could prevent the formation of sickle-shaped cells, thus reducing the disease's severity.

These strategies are still in the experimental stages, but clinical trials have already demonstrated significant success. Several patients have been treated with gene therapy and have shown remarkable improvement, with some achieving **normal red blood cell production** and experiencing **pain-free periods** for the first time in years. While these treatments are not without risk, and long-term effects are still being studied, gene therapy offers the possibility of a permanent cure, transforming the outlook for individuals with sickle cell disease.

Gene Therapy for Thalassemia: Reducing the Need for Transfusions

Thalassemia is another genetic blood disorder caused by mutations in the genes responsible for producing hemoglobin. Unlike sickle cell disease, which results in abnormally shaped red blood cells, thalassemia leads to a **deficiency in hemoglobin** production, resulting in anemia and a range of complications. For people with thalassemia, **blood transfusions** are the standard treatment, but the need for lifelong transfusions often leads to **iron overload**, which can cause damage to vital organs like the liver and heart.

Gene therapy for thalassemia aims to eliminate or reduce the need for blood transfusions by **correcting the genetic defect** in the patient's hemoglobin genes. Researchers are primarily focused on two strategies:

1. **Gene Editing to Correct the Mutations:** Similar to sickle cell disease, gene editing technologies like CRISPR are being explored as a way to directly correct the mutations in the genes that code for hemoglobin. The goal is to restore normal hemoglobin production in patients with thalassemia, reducing the need for blood transfusions and improving overall health.
2. **Gene Addition to Increase Hemoglobin Production:** Another approach is to introduce a **healthy copy of the hemoglobin gene** into the patient's cells, allowing the body to produce normal hemoglobin. This technique has shown promise in animal studies, and early trials in humans have also demonstrated positive results. By increasing the amount of functional hemoglobin in the body, this approach could reduce the reliance on blood transfusions and improve the quality of life for thalassemia patients.

Just like in sickle cell disease, clinical trials for thalassemia gene therapy have shown encouraging results. Many patients have been able to stop or reduce their reliance on blood transfusions after receiving gene therapy, and some have experienced improved hemoglobin levels and fewer symptoms related to anemia.

Challenges and Ethical Considerations in Gene Therapy

While the potential benefits of gene therapy are vast, there are also several challenges and ethical considerations that need to be addressed before it can be widely used as a treatment for blood disorders.

1. **Safety and Long-Term Effects:** One of the biggest concerns with gene therapy is the **safety** of the procedures. Gene editing techniques, while powerful, can sometimes have unintended effects, such as **off-target mutations** or **immune system reactions**. Ensuring that gene therapy is both **safe and effective** in the long term is critical before it can become a mainstream treatment option.
2. **Cost and Accessibility:** Gene therapy is a complex and expensive procedure, and the costs associated with the treatments can be prohibitively high. For patients in low-resource settings or in countries with limited access to advanced medical care, gene therapy may not be an accessible option unless efforts are made to reduce costs and increase availability. There is also the issue of **insurance coverage** for gene therapy, which may not be available for all patients.
3. **Ethical Concerns:** Gene therapy raises several ethical concerns, particularly with regard to its **germline** application—altering the genetic material in sperm or egg cells, which would then be passed on to future generations. While germline gene therapy holds great potential for preventing inherited diseases, it also raises questions about the potential for **genetic modification**, the **equity of access**, and the **long-term consequences** for humanity as a whole.

The Future of Gene Therapy for Blood Disorders

As gene therapy technologies continue to advance, the future looks incredibly promising for patients with **genetic blood disorders**. Researchers are making rapid strides in improving the precision, safety, and accessibility of these treatments. In the coming years, gene therapy could become a **standard** part of the treatment for diseases like sickle cell disease and thalassemia, offering patients the possibility of a permanent cure.

Moreover, the success of gene therapy for blood disorders is likely to have a ripple effect across the entire field of medicine. If gene therapy proves to be effective for blood disorders, it could pave the way for treating other inherited diseases, including **genetic cancers**, **neurodegenerative disorders**, and even **autoimmune diseases**.

Advancements in **gene editing** technologies, such as **CRISPR-Cas9**, are making gene therapy more precise, affordable, and widely applicable. At the same time, **immunotherapy** and **stem cell** research are also converging with gene therapy, offering even more promising possibilities for patients with blood disorders.

Conclusion

Gene therapy is undoubtedly one of the most exciting and transformative advancements in the field of medicine. For individuals living with blood disorders like sickle cell disease and thalassemia, gene therapy offers a **potential cure** that could eliminate the need for lifelong blood transfusions, reduce the risk of complications, and ultimately improve their quality of life. While challenges remain, the progress that has been made so far is nothing short of remarkable. In the years to come, gene therapy could become a **mainstream** treatment option for genetic blood disorders, changing the future of healthcare and offering hope to millions of patients around the world.

Chapter 42

The Promise of CRISPR in Hematology

In recent years, **CRISPR-Cas9**, a revolutionary gene-editing technology, has emerged as a game-changer in the world of genetics and medicine. With its precision, efficiency, and affordability, CRISPR is rapidly transforming the way we approach the treatment of genetic diseases. Among the many applications of CRISPR, its potential to treat **genetic blood disorders** stands out as one of the most promising and exciting developments in modern healthcare.

In this chapter, we will explore how **CRISPR** works, its potential to treat genetic blood disorders like **sickle cell disease** and **thalassemia**, and the ethical, scientific, and clinical challenges that need to be addressed before CRISPR-based therapies can be widely used in hematology.

Understanding CRISPR-Cas9: A Revolution in Gene Editing

CRISPR stands for **Clustered Regularly Interspaced Short Palindromic Repeats**, a term that refers to a segment of DNA that was discovered in bacteria. In bacteria, CRISPR acts as a form of immune defense, protecting the organism from viruses by storing snippets of viral DNA in its genome. The Cas9 protein, which stands for **CRISPR-associated protein 9**, acts as a molecular scissors, cutting DNA at precise locations to edit the genome.

What makes CRISPR so revolutionary is its ability to **target specific genes** and **edit them with extreme precision**. By introducing a piece of genetic material into the DNA of a living organism, scientists can either disable a faulty gene, correct a mutation, or even insert a new, healthy gene in its place. This targeted gene-editing process allows researchers to make alterations at the **genetic level**, offering a potential cure for inherited genetic disorders.

The simplicity and efficiency of CRISPR have opened up new possibilities for **gene therapy**, particularly for **blood disorders** caused by mutations in the genes that produce **hemoglobin** or other critical components of blood. By using CRISPR to directly modify the genes responsible for these conditions, researchers believe it may be possible to correct the underlying cause of diseases like **sickle cell disease**, **thalassemia**, and **hemophilia**.

CRISPR in Sickle Cell Disease: A Potential Cure

Sickle cell disease is one of the most devastating genetic blood disorders, affecting millions of people worldwide. It is caused by a mutation in the **hemoglobin gene**, leading to the production of abnormally shaped red blood cells. These sickle-shaped cells can obstruct blood flow, leading to severe pain, organ damage, and a range of life-threatening complications. While current treatments like blood transfusions and pain management help alleviate symptoms, there is no permanent cure for sickle cell disease.

The potential for **CRISPR** to treat sickle cell disease lies in its ability to directly edit the hemoglobin gene, fixing the mutation that causes the disease. There are several approaches being researched, including:

1. **Direct Gene Editing of Hemoglobin:** One approach involves using CRISPR-Cas9 to directly edit the **hemoglobin gene** in patients' cells. By **correcting** the mutation in the gene that produces sickle-shaped hemoglobin, CRISPR could restore normal red blood cell function, eliminating the symptoms of sickle cell disease. This approach involves extracting **hematopoietic stem cells** from the patient's bone marrow, editing the genes in the lab, and then reinfusing the corrected cells into the patient's bloodstream.
2. **Inducing Fetal Hemoglobin Production:** Another promising approach is to **reactivate fetal hemoglobin** production in adult patients. During fetal development, babies produce a type of hemoglobin known as **fetal hemoglobin (HbF)**, which is different from the adult version of hemoglobin (HbA) and has a lower tendency to sickle. In individuals with sickle cell disease, reactivating HbF production could reduce the amount of sickle-shaped hemoglobin in the body, thereby alleviating symptoms. CRISPR can be used to modify the genes involved in the production of HbF, turning on the fetal hemoglobin pathway and offering a potential treatment for sickle cell disease.

The initial results from clinical trials using CRISPR to treat sickle cell disease are promising. In 2019, a groundbreaking study reported that patients who underwent CRISPR-based therapy experienced a **complete resolution of symptoms**, with some no longer requiring regular blood transfusions. While these results are still in early stages, they represent a significant step forward in the quest for a cure for sickle cell disease.

CRISPR and Thalassemia: Correcting Hemoglobin Deficiency

Thalassemia is another genetic blood disorder that is characterized by a deficiency in hemoglobin production. Unlike sickle cell disease, which produces abnormally shaped red blood cells, thalassemia results in insufficient or faulty hemoglobin, leading to **anemia** and a variety of complications, including **iron overload** from frequent blood transfusions. In severe cases, individuals with thalassemia may require lifelong transfusions to survive.

Gene therapy using CRISPR offers a promising solution to thalassemia by **correcting the genetic mutations** that impair hemoglobin production. There are two main approaches being researched:

1. **Gene Editing to Correct the Mutation:** Just as with sickle cell disease, one approach involves using CRISPR to **directly edit** the genes responsible for producing defective hemoglobin in thalassemia patients. By repairing the mutations in the hemoglobin genes, it may be possible to restore normal hemoglobin production, reducing or eliminating the need for blood transfusions.
2. **Gene Addition to Boost Hemoglobin Levels:** Another approach is to use CRISPR to introduce a **functional copy of the hemoglobin gene** into the patient's genome. This could help boost the production of healthy hemoglobin, alleviating the symptoms of thalassemia and reducing the need for frequent transfusions.

In clinical trials, patients with beta-thalassemia who have undergone CRISPR-based treatments have shown **significant improvements** in hemoglobin levels and reduced dependency on blood transfusions. These promising results suggest that CRISPR could play a crucial role in the future treatment of thalassemia, offering a potential cure for individuals living with this chronic condition.

The Challenges and Ethical Considerations of CRISPR in Hematology

While CRISPR holds immense potential, its use in gene editing—particularly for blood disorders—comes with several **scientific, clinical, and ethical challenges**. Some of the key concerns include:

1. **Safety and Precision:** Although CRISPR is highly precise, there is still a risk of **off-target effects**, where the technology unintentionally alters genes that it was not meant to target. These unintended changes could lead to

adverse effects, such as the development of cancer or other health problems. Researchers are working diligently to improve the **accuracy** of CRISPR, but ensuring the safety of these treatments remains a priority.

2. **Long-Term Effects:** While early clinical trials have shown promising results, the long-term effects of CRISPR-based therapies are still largely unknown. Researchers are closely monitoring patients who have undergone gene editing to ensure that the treatment is not only effective but also safe in the long term. The possibility of **genetic modifications** being passed down to future generations also raises concerns about unintended consequences.

3. **Ethical and Social Implications:** CRISPR technology has the potential to alter the genetic makeup of future generations, which raises significant ethical questions. For example, **germline editing** (editing the genes of embryos or reproductive cells) could potentially lead to unintended changes in the gene pool, which may have far-reaching consequences for society. There are also concerns about **equity**—the accessibility of gene therapy for people in low-income regions, and whether these treatments will be available to all patients who need them.

4. **Cost and Accessibility:** Gene therapy using CRISPR is a complex and costly process, involving genetic modifications in laboratories, cell extraction, and reinfusion. As a result, the cost of CRISPR-based therapies could be prohibitive for many patients, particularly in low-income countries. Efforts are underway to reduce the costs of these treatments, but ensuring accessibility remains a challenge.

The Future of CRISPR in Hematology

Despite these challenges, the future of CRISPR-based gene therapy in the treatment of blood disorders is incredibly promising. The rapid advancement of gene-editing technologies and ongoing clinical trials offer hope that CRISPR could one day become a **mainstream treatment** for diseases like sickle cell disease and thalassemia. Researchers are continuing to refine the technology, improving its safety, efficiency, and precision.

In addition to its potential in hematology, CRISPR holds promise for the treatment of a wide range of genetic diseases, including **cancer, neurological disorders**, and **immune diseases**. As the technology matures, its impact on the field of medicine could be **transformational**, offering new hope for patients suffering from conditions that were once considered **untreatable**.

Conclusion

CRISPR-Cas9 has the potential to revolutionize the treatment of **genetic blood disorders**, offering the possibility of **curing diseases** like sickle cell disease and thalassemia. By precisely editing the genes responsible for these conditions, CRISPR may be able to restore normal blood cell production, reduce symptoms, and even eliminate the need for lifelong treatments like blood transfusions. While challenges remain, particularly with regards to safety, ethics, and accessibility, the promise of CRISPR in hematology is undeniable. As research continues to advance, **gene editing** may one day offer a cure for millions of patients around the world, transforming the future of blood disorder treatments forever.

Chapter 43

The Global Impact of Blood Disorders

Blood disorders, though often overlooked in global health discussions, affect millions of people worldwide and present significant challenges not only to the individuals living with these conditions but also to the healthcare systems attempting to address them. From **anemia** and **hemophilia** to **sickle cell disease** and **thalassemia**, blood disorders are a broad category of medical conditions that span different regions, economic statuses, and cultural contexts. The burden of these diseases is felt disproportionately across the world, and factors such as **geographic location**, **access to care**, **socioeconomic status**, and **public health infrastructures** all contribute to the stark **disparities** in the treatment and management of blood disorders.

In this chapter, we will explore how blood disorders are treated across different regions of the world, focusing on the **variability** in access to diagnosis, care, and treatment. We will also examine the disparities that exist between **developed** and **developing countries**, the role of **global health initiatives**, and the ongoing efforts to improve the care and treatment of blood disorders worldwide.

Prevalence of Blood Disorders Globally

Blood disorders are among the most widespread yet under-recognized health issues across the globe. According to the **World Health Organization (WHO)**, **anemia**, a condition in which there is a deficiency in red blood cells or hemoglobin, affects more than **2 billion people**, making it the most common blood disorder worldwide. The leading cause of anemia is **iron deficiency**, which can be exacerbated by poor diet, malnutrition, and chronic diseases.

Other blood disorders, such as **sickle cell disease, thalassemia**, and **hemophilia**, are equally pervasive but are more localized in their distribution. **Sickle cell disease** predominantly affects individuals of African, Mediterranean, and Middle Eastern descent, while **thalassemia** is more common in populations of Mediterranean, Southeast Asian, and Middle Eastern origin. **Hemophilia**, a genetic disorder that impairs the blood's ability to clot, is found worldwide but is most commonly seen in men, as it is an X-linked recessive disorder.

While these diseases are widespread, the level of care and **accessibility to treatment** can vary significantly based on geography, resources, and infrastructure. Understanding how these disorders are addressed around the world requires examining both the **global patterns** and the **local realities** of healthcare access.

Healthcare Disparities: Developed vs. Developing Countries

The disparity between **developed** and **developing** countries in terms of access to blood disorder treatment is stark. In **high-income countries**, individuals with blood disorders generally have access to advanced diagnostic tools, specialized treatments, and multidisciplinary healthcare teams. In these countries, there is widespread availability of essential medications like **iron supplements**, **blood transfusions**, and **genetic therapies** for disorders like sickle cell disease and thalassemia. Moreover, **bone marrow transplants, gene therapy**, and **CRISPR-based treatments** have opened up new doors for curing blood disorders, offering hope to patients who might otherwise have faced lifelong suffering.

For example, in the United States and Western Europe, **blood transfusions** and **iron chelation therapy** are common treatments for individuals with **thalassemia** and **sickle cell disease**, and the advent of gene therapy has provided a potentially life-altering treatment for individuals with sickle cell disease. Additionally, **advanced screening programs** for newborns allow for early diagnosis and immediate intervention, which can significantly improve long-term health outcomes for individuals with blood disorders.

However, in **low-income countries**, the situation is often much bleaker. Limited access to medical facilities, a lack of trained healthcare professionals, and insufficient availability of essential medications and treatments contribute to poor outcomes for people living with blood disorders. **Blood transfusions** may be scarce, **iron supplements** can be difficult to obtain, and **genetic testing** or advanced **diagnostic technologies** are often unavailable. Furthermore, many people living with **hemophilia, sickle cell disease**, or **thalassemia** in these regions face challenges in accessing the necessary healthcare due to **financial constraints, geographic barriers**, and the lack of adequate healthcare infrastructure.

In some parts of sub-Saharan Africa, where **sickle cell disease** is prevalent, there is often a **lack of awareness** about the disease, leading to delayed diagnoses and inadequate treatment. **Blood transfusions** and **pain management** are not always readily available, and **genetic counseling** and **preventative care** are scarce. Patients may be left with limited options, facing chronic pain and complications without adequate access to life-saving treatments.

Challenges in Access to Treatment

The lack of access to appropriate care is not solely a matter of financial inequality; it also involves issues related to **education**, **awareness**, and **cultural perceptions** of disease. In many parts of the world, blood disorders such as sickle cell disease are still seen as **mysterious** or even **taboo**, with individuals sometimes experiencing **stigma** and **discrimination** due to their condition. This can delay diagnosis, limit access to appropriate treatment, and increase the emotional toll on both patients and their families.

Another significant challenge is the **cost** of treatment. In high-income countries, the healthcare system may cover the costs of life-saving treatments like blood transfusions, medication, or gene therapy, but these treatments can be prohibitively expensive for individuals in low-income countries. The **cost of medications**, such as **iron chelators**, used to prevent iron overload from repeated blood transfusions, can be especially high. **Gene therapy** and **bone marrow transplants** are still emerging treatments that can cost hundreds of thousands of dollars, making them inaccessible to patients in lower-income regions.

In addition to the financial burden, logistical barriers can further exacerbate disparities. The **delivery of blood products** in developing countries may be hindered by inadequate storage facilities, unreliable transportation systems, and a lack of trained personnel to oversee blood collection and distribution. These logistical issues can result in shortages of essential resources, especially in rural or underserved areas.

Global Health Initiatives and Efforts to Bridge the Gap

Despite the many challenges, there have been significant strides made in **global health initiatives** aimed at addressing blood disorders, particularly in resource-limited settings. **International organizations**, **NGOs**, and **governments** have come together to address the disparities in care and improve outcomes for patients worldwide.

The **World Health Organization (WHO)** has played a crucial role in improving awareness of blood disorders and has implemented various programs to combat **iron deficiency anemia** and promote **blood donation**. WHO's efforts to enhance **public health education** and improve diagnostic capabilities have helped countries identify and manage blood disorders more effectively, particularly in rural or underserved populations.

Additionally, **international partnerships** between organizations like the **Sickle Cell Disease Association of America (SCDAA)**, the **Thalassemia International Federation (TIF)**, and regional health bodies have made strides in promoting **screening** programs and facilitating **blood donations** for transfusion-dependent patients. Programs aimed at **early detection** of blood disorders in newborns have been particularly successful in some parts of Africa and South Asia, helping to reduce the impact of these diseases on children and improving overall health outcomes.

Efforts to address **hemophilia** in developing countries are also making progress. Organizations like the **World Federation of Hemophilia (WFH)** work to ensure that patients with bleeding disorders have access to **clotting factor** replacement therapies. They also run training programs for healthcare professionals, improving the diagnosis and management of hemophilia in low-resource settings.

On the research front, advances in **gene therapy** and **CRISPR-based treatments** offer hope for **curing genetic blood disorders** like sickle cell disease and thalassemia. **Philanthropic organizations** and **corporations** are investing in global initiatives to make these therapies more affordable and accessible, though significant barriers remain, particularly around cost and logistics.

The Future of Global Blood Disorder Treatment

Looking ahead, the future of blood disorder treatment on a global scale hinge on several key factors:

1. **Innovation in Treatment Accessibility:** Advances in **telemedicine, mobile health apps,** and **affordable diagnostic tools** can improve access to care, especially in remote areas. Making genetic testing and treatment more accessible will be crucial in reducing the burden of genetic blood disorders.
2. **Education and Awareness:** Raising awareness about blood disorders, particularly in low-income countries, is essential for early diagnosis and effective management. **Public health campaigns** and **educational outreach** can empower communities to seek timely medical help and reduce the stigma associated with these conditions.

3. **Global Partnerships:** Increased cooperation between international organizations, governments, and the private sector is key to addressing the complex challenges of blood disorder treatment worldwide. **Resource sharing, funding,** and **collaboration** will be necessary to overcome the financial, logistical, and healthcare infrastructure barriers faced by low-income countries.

4. **Affordable and Sustainable Treatments:** The cost of gene therapy and other cutting-edge treatments must be reduced to make them accessible to patients in all parts of the world. This requires **collaboration between researchers, pharmaceutical companies,** and **government agencies** to create **affordable solutions** that can be scaled globally.

Conclusion

The impact of blood disorders is a global challenge that affects millions of individuals and families across different regions and socioeconomic backgrounds. While significant advances in diagnosis, treatment, and management have been made in high-income countries, much work remains to address the disparities in care that exist between developed and developing nations. By focusing on **global health initiatives**, improving **accessibility** to treatments, and fostering **international cooperation**, we can begin to bridge the gap in care and provide better outcomes for individuals living with blood disorders worldwide. The future of blood disorder treatment will rely on both **scientific innovation** and **global solidarity**, creating a world where no one is left behind in the fight against these devastating diseases.

Chapter 44

The Next Frontier: Immunotherapies for Blood Cancer

Blood cancers, including **leukemia, lymphoma,** and **myeloma,** represent some of the most challenging cancers to treat, with a history of aggressive treatments that often involve chemotherapy, radiation, and stem cell transplants. However, in recent years, **immunotherapy** has emerged as a revolutionary approach, offering new hope for patients with blood cancers. Immunotherapy harnesses the body's **immune system** to identify, attack, and destroy cancer cells, and its potential is transforming the way we approach the treatment of blood cancers.

In this chapter, we will explore the advances in immunotherapy for blood cancers, how it works, the different types of therapies currently in use, and the future potential of these treatments in revolutionizing cancer care.

Understanding Immunotherapy

Immunotherapy is a type of **cancer treatment** that works by stimulating or enhancing the body's **immune system** to recognize and fight cancer cells. Unlike traditional cancer treatments, such as chemotherapy, which kill both cancerous and healthy cells indiscriminately, immunotherapy aims to target only the cancer cells. The immune system plays a crucial role in defending the body against infections and diseases, including cancer, but sometimes it fails to recognize cancer cells as dangerous due to various mechanisms that cancer cells use to evade detection. Immunotherapy works by overcoming these mechanisms and enabling the immune system to attack the cancer more effectively.

The immune system consists of a complex network of cells, tissues, and organs that work together to protect the body. Key players in the immune system's response to cancer include **T cells, B cells, natural killer cells,** and other immune system proteins. Immunotherapy enhances the activity of these cells and proteins to specifically target the cancerous cells.

The primary strategies employed in immunotherapy for blood cancers include **checkpoint inhibitors, CAR-T cell therapy, monoclonal antibodies, cancer vaccines,** and **immune cytokine therapies.** Each approach offers different

Checkpoint Inhibitors: Unlocking the Immune Response

One of the most prominent classes of immunotherapies used in the treatment of blood cancers is **checkpoint inhibitors**. These drugs work by blocking the checkpoints that cancer cells use to evade detection by the immune system. In a normal immune response, immune cells, like **T cells**, are activated to attack foreign invaders, including cancer cells. However, cancer cells can develop mechanisms to "turn off" this immune response by binding to certain **checkpoint proteins** on T cells, such as **PD-1** or **CTLA-4**. This effectively prevents the immune system from attacking the cancer cells.

Checkpoint inhibitors block these proteins, allowing T cells to stay active and continue attacking cancer cells. Some of the most commonly used checkpoint inhibitors include **nivolumab** (Opdivo) and **pembrolizumab** (Keytruda), which target the PD-1 protein. These therapies have shown significant success in treating various blood cancers, including **Hodgkin lymphoma** and **non-Hodgkin lymphoma**. The **FDA** has approved checkpoint inhibitors for the treatment of these cancers, and clinical trials have demonstrated improved outcomes for patients who were previously resistant to traditional therapies.

Checkpoint inhibitors work particularly well in cancers that have high **mutational burdens** or that exhibit **immune evasion** strategies. For example, some types of **Hodgkin lymphoma** have a **high expression of PD-L1**, the ligand for PD-1, which makes them more responsive to checkpoint blockade. In contrast, other cancers, such as **chronic lymphocytic leukemia (CLL)**, may require combination therapies to achieve the best results.

CAR-T Cell Therapy: Engineering the Immune System

Another groundbreaking approach in immunotherapy for blood cancers is **CAR-T cell therapy** (Chimeric Antigen Receptor T-cell therapy). This personalized treatment involves genetically modifying a patient's own **T cells** to better recognize and attack cancer cells. The process starts by collecting T cells from the patient's blood through a procedure known as **apheresis**. These T cells are then genetically engineered in the laboratory to express a receptor (called a **chimeric antigen receptor**) that specifically targets an antigen found on the surface of cancer cells.

Once the T cells have been modified, they are infused back into the patient's body, where they are now equipped to recognize and destroy the cancer cells. CAR-T therapy has proven to be a game-changer in the treatment of blood cancers, especially **acute lymphoblastic leukemia (ALL)** and **non-Hodgkin lymphoma**. One of the key targets for CAR-T cell therapy is the protein **CD19**, which is expressed on the surface of **B cells**, including malignant B cells in conditions like **B-cell acute lymphoblastic leukemia (B-ALL)** and **diffuse large B-cell lymphoma (DLBCL)**.

The FDA has approved several CAR-T therapies for the treatment of blood cancers, including **Kymriah** (tisagenlecleucel) and **Yescarta** (axicabtagene ciloleucel). These treatments have shown remarkable success, especially in patients who have relapsed or are refractory to conventional therapies. Clinical trials have reported high remission rates, and many patients who were previously facing limited treatment options have experienced long-term remission after CAR-T cell therapy.

However, CAR-T therapy is not without its challenges. The process of modifying and re-infusing the T cells is complex, and not all patients respond to the therapy. Additionally, CAR-T therapy can cause serious side effects, including **cytokine release syndrome (CRS)**, where the immune system releases a large amount of cytokines into the bloodstream, leading to inflammation and potential organ damage. **Neurological effects** are also a concern, and careful monitoring is required during treatment.

Despite these challenges, CAR-T therapy represents a significant breakthrough, offering a new hope for patients who previously had few options.

Monoclonal Antibodies: Targeting Cancer Cells Directly

Monoclonal antibodies (mAbs) are another form of immunotherapy that has been used successfully to treat blood cancers. These lab-made molecules are designed to mimic the immune system's ability to fight off harmful pathogens and cancer cells. Monoclonal antibodies work by targeting specific proteins on the surface of cancer cells, effectively marking them for destruction by the immune system.

For example, **rituximab** (Rituxan) is a monoclonal antibody that targets the **CD20** protein found on the surface of **B cells**. Rituximab has been widely used to treat **non-Hodgkin lymphoma** and **chronic lymphocytic leukemia (CLL)**. By binding to CD20, rituximab helps the immune system recognize and destroy the B cells that are cancerous. It can also be used in combination with chemotherapy or other immunotherapies to enhance its effectiveness.

Other monoclonal antibodies, such as **daratumumab** (Darzalex) and **isatuximab** (Sarclisa), target **CD38**, a protein that is overexpressed on the surface of **myeloma cells**. These therapies have shown significant promise in treating **multiple myeloma**, a cancer of the plasma cells in the bone marrow.

Monoclonal antibodies can be used as standalone treatments or in combination with other therapies, providing flexibility in how they are incorporated into treatment regimens. They are often well-tolerated, although side effects such as **infusion reactions** and **immune suppression** can occur.

Cancer Vaccines: Harnessing the Immune System's Potential

Another emerging area of immunotherapy is the use of **cancer vaccines**. Unlike traditional vaccines that are designed to prevent infection, **cancer vaccines** are intended to **treat** cancer by stimulating the immune system to attack cancer cells. These vaccines are often used in blood cancers like **leukemia**, **lymphoma**, and **myeloma**, where the goal is to activate the immune system to target and destroy cancer cells that express certain tumor-specific antigens.

One example of a cancer vaccine used in blood cancers is the **BCG vaccine** (Bacillus Calmette-Guérin), which is used in some clinical trials to treat **bladder cancer** and has been explored in combination with other therapies for blood cancers. Although cancer vaccines are still largely experimental, they hold great promise in the future treatment landscape, particularly as more is learned about the **tumor microenvironment** and how to manipulate it to benefit patients.

The Future of Immunotherapy for Blood Cancers

The future of immunotherapy for blood cancers is extremely promising. Ongoing research is focused on improving the effectiveness of existing therapies, expanding their use to a wider range of blood cancers, and reducing side effects. As scientists continue to explore the molecular and genetic basis of these diseases, more precise treatments can be developed to target cancer cells more effectively while minimizing damage to healthy tissue.

Emerging treatments like **bispecific antibodies**, which can target two different antigens simultaneously, and **immune checkpoint inhibitors** combined with **CAR-T therapies** are already showing promise in preclinical studies and early-phase clinical trials. Furthermore, advancements in **genomic sequencing** and **precision medicine** will allow for more tailored and personalized approaches, ensuring that patients receive the most appropriate treatment for their specific cancer type.

Immunotherapies are likely to play an increasing role in combination treatments, where they may work alongside traditional therapies like chemotherapy, radiation, and stem cell transplants to improve patient outcomes. These **combination strategies** hold the potential to enhance the efficacy of immunotherapies and overcome the resistance mechanisms that sometimes develop in cancer cells.

Chapter 45

The Role of Blood Banks in Saving Lives

Blood is an essential component of the human body, playing a vital role in transporting oxygen and nutrients, fighting infections, and maintaining overall health. Yet, for individuals facing blood disorders or those undergoing surgeries, cancer treatments, or accidents, the need for blood becomes even more critical. This is where **blood banks** come into play, playing a crucial role in ensuring that an adequate supply of blood is available for those in need.

In this chapter, we explore the operational dynamics of blood banks, the significance of blood donation, and how blood banks specifically help individuals suffering from blood disorders.

Understanding Blood Banks

A blood bank is a facility that collects, tests, processes, stores, and distributes blood and its components, such as plasma, red blood cells, and platelets, to hospitals and clinics. Blood banks serve as an essential lifeline for patients suffering from various medical conditions, including **blood disorders**, trauma, major surgeries, and certain chronic illnesses. These facilities work closely with healthcare systems, providing a critical supply of blood to support life-saving treatments.

The process within blood banks involves several key stages: collection, screening, processing, testing, and distribution. Let's examine each step:

1. **Blood Collection**: Blood collection occurs in various settings, including **donation centers**, **mobile blood drives**, and **hospitals**. Donors are typically volunteers who give blood on a regular basis. The collection process is relatively simple and typically takes about 10 minutes for whole blood donation, during which one unit (approximately 450 milliliters) of blood is drawn. Some blood centers may also collect specific components, like platelets or plasma, depending on the needs of the recipients.
2. **Screening and Testing**: After collection, donated blood undergoes rigorous screening for **infectious diseases** such as HIV, hepatitis B, and hepatitis C, among others. Blood banks also test for blood type (A, B, AB, O) and Rh factor (positive or negative). This is essential to ensure that the donated

blood is compatible with the recipient's blood type, reducing the risk of adverse reactions during transfusions.

3. **Processing**: Once blood is tested, it is processed into its individual components—**red blood cells, plasma, platelets**, and **cryoprecipitate**. Red blood cells are primarily used for treating anemia and significant blood loss, plasma is used for clotting disorders and burns, platelets help patients with blood clotting disorders, and cryoprecipitate is used in treating bleeding disorders. Processing allows for a more targeted approach in meeting the specific needs of patients, ensuring efficient and effective treatment.

4. **Storage and Distribution**: Blood components are stored in specialized refrigeration units, with red blood cells typically stored for up to **42 days**, while platelets are stored at room temperature for up to **five days**. Plasma can be frozen and stored for extended periods. Blood banks maintain strict protocols to ensure the integrity and safety of blood products before they are distributed to hospitals and healthcare facilities.

The Importance of Blood Donation

Blood donation is the cornerstone of the blood banking system, as without donations, blood banks would be unable to provide life-saving blood supplies to those in need. There are many reasons why people donate blood, and understanding these motivations helps underscore the importance of maintaining a healthy blood supply.

- **Life-Saving Need**: For individuals with **blood disorders** such as **anemia, hemophilia,** or **sickle cell disease**, blood donations are often crucial for managing their condition. For instance, individuals with sickle cell disease may require regular blood transfusions to manage pain, prevent strokes, and reduce the severity of symptoms. Similarly, people with anemia caused by **iron deficiency, vitamin B12 deficiency**, or chronic diseases might need red blood cell transfusions to correct low hemoglobin levels.
- **Emergencies and Trauma**: In cases of accidents, surgeries, or trauma, blood transfusions are often required to replace lost blood. For instance, patients undergoing **major surgeries** such as heart bypass operations, organ transplants, or cancer treatments often lose significant amounts of blood and may require blood transfusions to maintain their life-sustaining bodily functions. Blood banks are essential in providing the necessary support during these high-risk procedures.
- **Chronic Conditions**: Patients with **leukemia, lymphoma,** or **myeloma** often rely on blood transfusions, platelets, and other blood components

during their treatment. Chemotherapy and radiation therapies, which are common treatments for blood cancers, can suppress the production of blood cells and lower platelet counts, increasing the need for transfusions. Blood banks play an essential role in ensuring that these patients can undergo treatment without the additional complication of blood deficiencies.

- **Cancer Treatment**: Blood transfusions, particularly red blood cell transfusions and platelet infusions, are vital for patients undergoing **chemotherapy** or **radiation therapy**. These treatments can significantly impact the production of blood cells in the bone marrow, leading to **anemia** and **low platelet counts**. In such cases, blood bank supplies are critical to help patients maintain their treatment schedule and recovery.
- **Emergencies and Natural Disasters**: Blood donation also plays a key role during natural disasters, such as earthquakes, hurricanes, or other emergencies. When large numbers of people are injured, there is often a sudden surge in the demand for blood, and blood banks are on the front lines in providing this critical resource. The preparedness of blood banks to respond to emergencies is a testament to the importance of regular blood donations.

Blood Banks and Their Role in Blood Disorder Management

For individuals with chronic blood disorders like **sickle cell disease, thalassemia**, and **hemophilia**, blood transfusions from blood banks are sometimes needed on a regular basis. These individuals often rely on **blood donations** to maintain their health and manage the complications associated with their conditions. Blood banks become crucial partners in the care of these patients, ensuring that they have access to the appropriate type of blood or blood component when needed.

For example, **sickle cell disease** is a genetic condition that leads to the production of abnormally shaped red blood cells, which can cause blockages in blood vessels, pain, and organ damage. Regular blood transfusions can help reduce the number of sickle-shaped cells and improve blood flow. Similarly, individuals with **thalassemia**, a genetic disorder that causes an imbalance in hemoglobin production, often require lifelong blood transfusions to compensate for the lack of healthy red blood cells.

For patients with **hemophilia**, a bleeding disorder where the blood doesn't clot properly, blood banks provide platelets and clotting factor concentrates. Hemophilia patients can experience frequent and spontaneous bleeding episodes, and access to these critical components is vital for managing the disease. Blood banks work closely with **specialized hematologists** and care teams to ensure that hemophilia patients have the resources they need for effective treatment.

The Role of Blood Banks in Advancing Research and Treatment

In addition to providing essential blood products to patients, blood banks are also deeply involved in the research and development of new treatments for blood disorders. The blood donated by individuals can be used in clinical research to better understand the underlying causes of blood disorders, improve transfusion practices, and develop new therapies. Blood banks work in partnership with **research institutions**, **hospitals**, and **pharmaceutical companies** to advance medical knowledge and improve patient care.

Blood banks also play a role in the development of blood substitutes, which are an area of active research. Artificial blood or synthetic blood, designed to perform some of the functions of natural blood, holds promise for addressing blood shortages and providing a viable option for patients who cannot receive conventional blood transfusions. The research efforts in this area depend on the expertise of blood banks to provide samples and test new blood-related products.

Challenges in Blood Donation and Supply

While blood banks play an essential role in healthcare, they face a number of challenges, particularly in maintaining a sufficient blood supply. One of the primary obstacles is the **shortage of blood donors**. Despite the fact that **one in seven hospital patients** will need a blood transfusion, the demand often exceeds the supply. This is particularly problematic during holidays or times when fewer people donate, which can lead to critical shortages.

Additionally, not everyone is eligible to donate blood due to various health conditions, such as **chronic illnesses**, **infectious diseases**, or **recent surgeries**. This creates a gap between the supply and demand for blood donations, making it even more important to encourage regular donations from healthy individuals.

Moreover, **blood donation awareness** remains a critical issue. Despite widespread efforts to educate the public about the importance of blood donation, there is still a significant lack of knowledge and understanding about the life-saving role of blood donation. Blood banks and advocacy organizations continue to work to increase public awareness and ensure a stable blood supply for those in need.

Conclusion

Blood banks are indispensable in the fight against blood disorders and in saving lives across the globe. Their ability to collect, process, test, store, and distribute blood components ensures that patients facing life-threatening conditions or undergoing treatments have the support they need. The role of **blood donation** cannot be overstated—it is a selfless act that directly impacts the lives of individuals suffering from **blood disorders** and those in critical need of transfusions.

As medical technology continues to advance and research into alternative blood products progresses, the importance of blood banks and **donor participation** in saving lives remains as relevant as ever. Through continued education, research, and efforts to boost donor participation, blood banks will continue to play a central role in healthcare and in ensuring that no patient has to face a shortage of blood during their time of need.

Chapter 46

Living Beyond the Blood

Living with a blood disorder can be an overwhelming experience, characterized by daily management, medical treatments, and the unpredictable nature of flare-ups. However, it is also possible to thrive despite these challenges. Thriving with a blood disorder is not just about surviving—it's about embracing a holistic approach to health that incorporates physical, emotional, and social well-being. This chapter explores the importance of maintaining a balance between medical care, self-care, emotional resilience, and community support. It highlights how individuals can take charge of their health, foster meaningful connections, and lead fulfilling lives, beyond the limitations of their condition.

Embracing the Body, Mind, and Spirit

While managing a blood disorder often involves regular medical care, treatments, and symptom management, true well-being requires attention to all aspects of a person's life. **Holistic health** means caring for the whole person—not just focusing on the physical symptoms of a blood disorder, but also nurturing mental and emotional health.

Physical Health and Lifestyle Choices

Physical health for someone with a blood disorder can sometimes be a delicate balance. Certain conditions, like **sickle cell disease** or **hemophilia**, can lead to chronic pain, fatigue, and limited physical ability. However, staying active and maintaining a healthy lifestyle is crucial for managing symptoms and improving overall quality of life.

1. **Dietary Choices:** Nutrition plays a critical role in supporting the body's natural healing processes. For individuals with blood disorders such as anemia, ensuring an adequate intake of nutrients like iron, folate, and vitamin B12 is essential. These nutrients are crucial for red blood cell production and overall energy levels. A balanced diet rich in fruits, vegetables, lean proteins, and whole grains can help manage symptoms and prevent complications.
2. **Exercise:** Physical activity, when tailored to individual needs, can be beneficial for those living with blood disorders. For example, **gentle**

exercises such as walking, yoga, swimming, or cycling can help improve circulation, reduce fatigue, and manage pain. Regular physical activity also boosts mental health by releasing endorphins, which are natural mood boosters. It's important for individuals to consult with their healthcare provider to determine which types of exercise are best suited for their condition.

3. **Managing Pain and Fatigue:** For those living with conditions like **sickle cell disease** or **beta-thalassemia**, pain and fatigue are common challenges. Regular pain management, whether through medication or alternative therapies like acupuncture, can help improve quality of life. Ensuring adequate rest is also important, as fatigue is a common symptom of many blood disorders. Creating a routine that includes rest and relaxation is key to managing energy levels.

4. **Preventive Healthcare:** Regular check-ups, blood tests, and screenings are essential for preventing complications and monitoring the progression of the condition. Early detection of any changes in blood health can prevent more serious issues down the line. Preventive care can also involve vaccinations or other treatments to manage associated conditions.

Emotional Well-Being: Navigating the Mental Health Landscape

Living with a blood disorder is not only physically demanding but can also take a significant toll on emotional well-being. Chronic illness can bring about feelings of frustration, sadness, isolation, and stress. These emotions, if left unchecked, can affect the body's ability to heal and manage symptoms effectively. Therefore, **mental health care** is a fundamental part of holistic health.

1. **Coping with Anxiety and Depression:** Individuals with chronic illnesses, such as blood disorders, often experience heightened levels of anxiety and depression. These mental health issues can be exacerbated by concerns about the future, treatment options, and social stigma. **Psychological support**—including therapy, counseling, and support groups—can help individuals process these feelings. Cognitive-behavioral therapy (CBT), for example, helps individuals manage negative thought patterns that might arise in response to their condition.

2. **Mindfulness and Stress Reduction:** Mindfulness practices, such as meditation, deep breathing, and mindfulness-based stress reduction (MBSR), can help individuals living with blood disorders cope with daily stress. These practices can help reduce anxiety, improve focus, and promote

relaxation, which can, in turn, improve physical health by lowering blood pressure and reducing inflammation.

3. **Building Emotional Resilience:** Developing emotional resilience is crucial for managing the emotional challenges of living with a blood disorder. Resilience allows individuals to face challenges with a positive mindset, adapt to changes, and maintain hope. Building emotional resilience can be done through practices like **gratitude journaling**, engaging in positive self-talk, and setting realistic goals.

4. **Self-Care and Relaxation:** Engaging in self-care activities that bring joy and relaxation can help manage stress and improve mental well-being. This might include hobbies such as reading, art, gardening, or spending time with loved ones. Setting aside time for relaxation—whether it's through a warm bath, a nap, or spending time outdoors—can also help individuals recharge and cope with the emotional demands of living with a chronic condition.

Community Support: Connecting with Others

One of the most powerful ways to thrive with a blood disorder is through the support of a **community**. No one should have to face the challenges of living with a blood disorder alone, and having a strong network of family, friends, healthcare providers, and peers can make all the difference. **Support systems** can provide practical help, emotional encouragement, and a sense of belonging.

1. **Family and Friends:** The support of family and friends is invaluable. Open communication with loved ones can help ease the burden of a blood disorder. These individuals can offer emotional support, assist with daily tasks, and accompany patients to medical appointments. However, it's also important for family members and friends to take care of their own emotional well-being to avoid burnout. Encouraging loved ones to access their own support networks, such as counseling or support groups, can strengthen the entire family system.

2. **Peer Support Groups:** Connecting with others who share similar experiences is one of the most effective ways to combat feelings of isolation. **Peer support groups**—whether in person or online—allow individuals with blood disorders to share their experiences, learn coping strategies, and find strength in the knowledge that they are not alone. Peer groups often provide a sense of camaraderie and solidarity that is uniquely comforting.

3. **Healthcare Providers as Part of the Support Team:** Healthcare providers play a critical role in a patient's journey. A compassionate and knowledgeable healthcare team—consisting of doctors, nurses, counselors,

and social workers—can help individuals navigate the medical aspects of living with a blood disorder. A strong patient-provider relationship based on trust and understanding helps individuals feel empowered in their treatment choices. Healthcare providers can also guide patients in connecting with support groups and community resources.

4. **Advocacy and Awareness:** Being part of the broader advocacy and awareness movement can also provide a sense of purpose and connection. Many individuals find that participating in awareness campaigns, fundraising efforts, or research initiatives gives them a voice in a world where blood disorders are often misunderstood. Advocacy work can provide a sense of empowerment and a chance to help educate others, thus reducing stigma and raising awareness about the challenges faced by individuals with blood disorders.

Finding Meaning Beyond the Illness

Living with a blood disorder often requires a shift in perspective. While it can be a source of stress and frustration, it can also lead to profound personal growth. For many, their experience with chronic illness offers an opportunity to connect with others, find strength in vulnerability, and redefine what it means to live a meaningful life.

Living beyond the blood is about recognizing that a blood disorder does not define who you are. It is possible to pursue passions, foster relationships, and contribute to society while managing a chronic condition. Whether through work, volunteering, creative expression, or simply spending time with loved ones, there are countless ways to find fulfillment.

At its core, living beyond the blood is about embracing a life of balance—managing the demands of the condition while also cherishing the joys of life. It's about cultivating **resilience**, **hope**, and **purpose**, regardless of the challenges posed by a blood disorder.

Conclusion

Thrive, rather than simply survive—this is the message for individuals living with blood disorders. The journey may be difficult, but with the right tools, support, and mindset, individuals can find joy and fulfillment in life. Holistic health, emotional resilience, and community support are essential components of thriving, and they are available to all. With a focus on self-care, emotional well-being, and building strong relationships, individuals with blood disorders can go beyond their condition and live lives filled with purpose, strength, and hope.

Chapter 47

Redefining What It Means to Be Healthy

Health is often seen as a simple equation—absence of disease, physical strength, mental clarity, and overall vitality. For most people, health is associated with the idea of being physically fit, mentally stable, and free from illness. However, living with a blood disorder challenges these traditional perceptions and calls for a more nuanced and inclusive definition of health. Blood disorders, whether inherited or acquired, affect not only the body but also the way individuals view themselves and interact with the world around them. This chapter explores how living with a blood disorder challenges conventional ideas of health, wellness, and normalcy, and how embracing a broader perspective on health can lead to a more compassionate, understanding, and inclusive society.

Health Beyond the Physical Body

When society talks about health, the focus is often on physical appearance and the ability to perform daily tasks without interruption. The emphasis is placed on **vitality, fitness, and strength**, but for individuals living with blood disorders like **sickle cell anemia**, **hemophilia**, or **thalassemia**, their experiences redefine what health truly means. These conditions don't always manifest in ways that are visible to others. They are often invisible diseases, and their effects can be sporadic— flare-ups may come and go, making it hard to pinpoint a concrete moment of illness or wellness.

1. **Chronic Illness and Visibility:** In a society where health is often equated with how one looks or how easily one moves, individuals with chronic blood disorders may not fit the mold of what is considered "healthy." Blood disorders like anemia or sickle cell disease often present with periods of wellness interspersed with bouts of pain, fatigue, or other complications. This variability challenges the common notion that health is a static state that can be visibly measured. Those living with these conditions might appear outwardly healthy yet struggle with constant, invisible challenges that require ongoing management.
2. **Health and Functionality:** For individuals with blood disorders, health isn't always about physical strength or the ability to perform the same tasks as those without illness. It's about finding ways to function within the limitations imposed by their condition. For example, someone with

hemophilia may need to carefully manage their physical activity to avoid bleeding episodes, while someone with **iron-deficiency anemia** might need to monitor their energy levels and adjust their routine accordingly. These individuals redefine what it means to be "fit" and focus on function over perfection.

3. **Pain as a Part of Health:** Pain, whether chronic or episodic, is an integral part of life for many individuals living with blood disorders. For those with **sickle cell disease**, frequent pain crises can leave them bedridden, while those with **thrombosis** or **hemophilia** may face bleeding episodes that lead to discomfort and long recovery periods. In this context, health is not simply about being free of pain or discomfort—it is about managing and coping with pain in ways that allow individuals to maintain their sense of self and continue pursuing their goals. This shift in understanding asks society to recognize that the absence of pain doesn't equate to the presence of health. Health can coexist with pain and chronic illness.

Mental and Emotional Wellness: A Hidden Aspect of Health

While physical health has long been the central focus in societal perceptions of well-being, emotional and mental health is often overlooked—especially for individuals with chronic blood disorders. The mental toll of living with a lifelong condition can be as debilitating as the physical symptoms, yet mental health is frequently underestimated in discussions about overall wellness.

1. **Psychological Impact of Chronic Illness:** The psychological effects of living with a blood disorder are vast. The constant management of health, frequent medical appointments, and the uncertainty about flare-ups can lead to feelings of stress, anxiety, and depression. For some, the emotional burden of knowing that their health is unpredictable can be overwhelming. This underscores the importance of recognizing that mental health is a crucial component of overall wellness. By integrating mental health care into the treatment of blood disorders, individuals can better manage not only their physical symptoms but also their emotional and psychological well-being.

2. **Stigma and Self-Perception:** Living with a blood disorder can sometimes lead to feelings of isolation, shame, or frustration, especially if the condition is misunderstood or stigmatized. Societal attitudes about health can perpetuate feelings of inadequacy in individuals who do not meet the conventional "healthy" standard. The stigma surrounding certain blood disorders, such as **sickle cell disease** or **hemophilia**, can lead to

discrimination or social isolation. Overcoming these barriers requires a shift in societal attitudes that sees health as more than just physical vitality—it is also about emotional resilience, the capacity to adapt, and the willingness to accept and support those living with health challenges.

3. **Redefining Success and Wellness:** Health, in the context of blood disorders, is also about redefining what it means to be successful and well. It's about managing a condition while still pursuing personal goals, achieving small victories, and maintaining relationships. It's about taking control over one's health through lifestyle choices, self-care, and emotional support. Success is no longer measured by the absence of disease but by the ability to live a fulfilling life despite challenges. This definition of wellness allows individuals to find joy, meaning, and purpose beyond their blood disorder.

Social Perceptions and the Need for Inclusion

Society's perception of health is heavily influenced by cultural norms and ideals, which often prioritize individuals who fit the physical "ideal" of health. However, those living with blood disorders challenge these conventional notions and demand a broader understanding of what it means to be healthy.

1. **Visibility and Awareness:** Increasing awareness about the wide variety of blood disorders and their impact on individuals' lives is crucial. Many blood disorders are underreported, misunderstood, or stigmatized. Conditions like **hemophilia, sickle cell disease**, and **anemia** don't always show visible signs, leading to misconceptions that these disorders are less serious than they truly are. It is vital for society to move away from focusing solely on appearance or "perfect health" and embrace a more inclusive understanding of wellness. This shift requires education, increased visibility, and advocacy, all of which can help foster a society that is more compassionate and accepting of those with chronic health conditions.

2. **Workplace and Social Integration:** The impact of blood disorders extends to all areas of life, including the workplace, schools, and social environments. People with blood disorders may need accommodations to manage their condition—whether it's flexible working hours, physical adaptations in the workplace, or understanding from peers and colleagues. Challenging the notion that only "healthy" individuals can contribute meaningfully to society requires a collective effort to create more inclusive spaces where people living with chronic conditions can thrive. **Policies** that promote inclusion, reduce stigma, and support individuals in all aspects of

their lives will help ensure that people with blood disorders can live without fear of exclusion or discrimination.

3. **Shifting Perspectives on Wellness:** Wellness should not be limited to physical health alone—it is a multifaceted concept that encompasses mental, emotional, and social well-being. For individuals with blood disorders, wellness is about achieving balance in these areas. **Holistic health** practices that focus on the whole person, including their physical, emotional, and mental state, should be normalized in discussions about health. By expanding the definition of wellness, society can move toward a more inclusive model where everyone, regardless of their physical condition, has the opportunity to lead a fulfilling and meaningful life.

Conclusion

Living with a blood disorder forces a reevaluation of what health truly means. It challenges the physical-centric narrative that dominates modern discussions of wellness and advocates for a broader, more inclusive perspective. By recognizing the importance of emotional resilience, social inclusion, and the need for holistic care, society can begin to redefine health as a dynamic and multifaceted concept—one that goes beyond physical appearance and functionality.

Those living with blood disorders offer valuable insight into the complexity of health and wellness. They prove that health is not simply the absence of disease but the ability to adapt, thrive, and find meaning in life despite adversity. By embracing this broader understanding of health, society can work toward creating a more compassionate and inclusive world where everyone, regardless of their health status, is empowered to live a full, meaningful life.

Chapter 48

The Power of Education and Awareness

Blood disorders, whether rare or common, invisible or apparent, are a crucial aspect of healthcare that demands greater visibility, understanding, and attention. From the genetic inheritance of conditions like **sickle cell anemia** and **thalassemia** to the acquired challenges of **hemophilia** and **anemia**, these conditions affect millions of people worldwide. However, despite their prevalence and severity, many blood disorders are poorly understood by the general public, healthcare providers, and even policymakers. This gap in knowledge can lead to delays in diagnosis, improper treatments, stigmatization, and, ultimately, a diminished quality of life for those affected. The transformative power of education and awareness is a key driver in improving the lives of individuals with blood disorders, and in this chapter, we explore why it is critical to educate and raise awareness about these life-altering conditions.

The Need for Public Education: Breaking the Silence

In many societies, blood disorders are misunderstood or even invisible to the public eye. Rare genetic conditions like **hemophilia** or **sickle cell disease** often go undiagnosed for years, and individuals living with these disorders can experience difficulty in accessing care and support. The absence of awareness is not just a problem in the general public; it also permeates social systems, schools, workplaces, and communities, where misconceptions and lack of understanding can lead to negative consequences such as discrimination, isolation, and missed opportunities for early intervention.

1. **Addressing Stigma and Misconceptions:** The stigma surrounding blood disorders, especially **sickle cell anemia** and **hemophilia**, often stems from a lack of knowledge and understanding. For instance, sickle cell disease is frequently mistaken for a condition that only affects certain racial or ethnic groups, leading to harmful stereotypes and social marginalization. By promoting education, the public can better understand that these conditions are not defined by race, and that anyone can be affected by them, regardless of background. Similarly, **hemophilia** is often misunderstood as a rare or

isolated condition, but in fact, it affects people all over the world and has significant health and social implications.

2. **Raising Awareness in Schools and Communities:** Children with blood disorders often face significant challenges in schools due to a lack of understanding from teachers, peers, and even healthcare staff. For example, children with **hemophilia** might be at risk for bleeding due to minor injuries, and if school personnel are unaware of this, it could lead to life-threatening situations. By educating schools and community organizations about the unique needs of students with blood disorders, we can ensure that these individuals receive the accommodations, care, and respect they need to thrive. Education can help people recognize the invisible challenges that others may face and foster greater empathy and understanding in communities.

3. **Understanding Chronic Conditions and Invisible Illnesses:** Many blood disorders, such as **iron-deficiency anemia, vitamin B12 deficiency**, and **chronic kidney disease-related anemia,** may not have outward symptoms or physical markers. This makes them easy to overlook or misinterpret, both by the public and sometimes by healthcare providers. In many cases, individuals may look perfectly healthy on the outside, yet still experience debilitating symptoms like chronic fatigue, dizziness, or shortness of breath. Educating the public about these "invisible" illnesses can reduce misunderstandings and help others offer the necessary support to those affected.

Healthcare Provider Education: Empowering the Frontlines

Healthcare providers, including doctors, nurses, and emergency medical professionals, are the first line of defense in diagnosing and treating blood disorders. However, despite the prevalence of these conditions, **blood disorders are often under-recognized, misdiagnosed, or mismanaged** in clinical settings. This lack of awareness among healthcare professionals can lead to delayed diagnoses, incorrect treatments, and unnecessary suffering for patients. For healthcare providers, continued education on the latest advancements, diagnostic techniques, and treatment options is paramount in improving the care of individuals living with blood disorders.

1. **Training and Knowledge on Rare Blood Disorders:** Conditions like **hemophilia, thalassemia,** and **sickle cell anemia** may be rare, but they are not rare enough to be ignored. Healthcare providers need to be equipped with the knowledge to identify symptoms and understand the intricacies of

these disorders. Continuing medical education (CME) programs and updated curricula in medical schools can help future generations of healthcare professionals recognize the signs of blood disorders early, make informed decisions, and offer the most appropriate treatments.

2. **Improved Diagnostic Tools and Protocols:** Early detection of blood disorders can significantly improve the quality of life for individuals, yet many conditions are not diagnosed until later stages. Diagnostic protocols and screening tests for certain blood disorders should be a part of routine healthcare, particularly in high-risk populations. Educating healthcare providers about the importance of early screening and providing them with updated diagnostic tools can lead to quicker identification and more effective treatment plans.

3. **Specialized Care and Multidisciplinary Approaches:** Managing blood disorders often requires a collaborative, multidisciplinary approach that involves not only hematologists but also primary care doctors, dietitians, pain specialists, psychologists, and other healthcare professionals. Education about blood disorders should extend beyond hematologists to include professionals across various medical fields. For example, educating **physical therapists** and **rehabilitation specialists** about the impact of **hemophilia** or **sickle cell disease** on mobility and physical activity can help improve patient outcomes. In turn, having a holistic, multidisciplinary care approach improves the overall management of the condition.

4. **Culturally Sensitive Care:** Blood disorders are often linked to genetic predispositions, and many conditions disproportionately affect specific populations or ethnic groups. **Sickle cell anemia**, for example, is most common in people of African, Mediterranean, Middle Eastern, and Indian descent. **Thalassemia** predominantly affects individuals of Mediterranean, Middle Eastern, and Southeast Asian backgrounds. Healthcare providers must be educated on the cultural, social, and genetic factors that influence these diseases in order to provide better, more personalized care. Culturally sensitive education programs can reduce biases, enhance patient-provider communication, and ensure that care is inclusive and equitable for all patients, regardless of their background.

Policy Makers and Public Health Advocacy: Creating Change

Policymakers and public health officials have a profound role to play in raising awareness and funding for blood disorder research, treatment, and education. In many countries, the management of blood disorders is still underfunded or poorly integrated into national healthcare systems, and patients often face barriers to accessing life-saving treatments. As such, it is critical to **advocate for policy change** that addresses the needs of individuals with blood disorders and ensures that appropriate resources are allocated toward education, research, and care.

1. **Research Funding and Access to Treatment:** Adequate funding for research into blood disorders is essential for developing new, innovative treatments and potential cures. Policymakers must prioritize funding for **genetic research, blood transfusion safety, stem cell therapies**, and **new drug developments**. Without sufficient investment in research, progress will stagnate, and patients may not have access to the latest treatment options. Furthermore, ensuring that these treatments are accessible to all populations—regardless of socioeconomic status, race, or geographic location—is key to achieving health equity in the management of blood disorders.

2. **Creating National Screening Programs:** Governments should consider implementing national or regional screening programs for blood disorders, especially in populations at high risk. Early detection can prevent complications, reduce healthcare costs in the long term, and improve the quality of life for individuals. Policymakers can take steps to ensure that **universal screening** for conditions like **sickle cell disease** and **thalassemia** is available as part of routine healthcare.

3. **Public Awareness Campaigns:** Governments and nonprofit organizations can collaborate to create public health campaigns that raise awareness about blood disorders. These campaigns can provide essential information about symptoms, risk factors, and treatment options. They can also address misconceptions and educate the public on how they can support those affected by blood disorders. Advocacy can help reduce stigma, encourage early diagnosis, and ensure that those affected by blood disorders receive the care and respect they deserve.

Conclusion

Education is a powerful tool that can break down barriers, eliminate stigma, and foster empathy and understanding. For individuals with blood disorders, education and awareness are not just about improving public knowledge; they are about improving quality of life, expanding access to care, and ensuring that every patient is treated with the dignity and respect they deserve. **Healthcare providers, policymakers**, and **the general public** must work together to foster a more inclusive and informed society—one where blood disorders are no longer a source of confusion, fear, or discrimination, but an area of knowledge, compassion, and support.

By investing in education and raising awareness, we not only improve the lives of those living with blood disorders, but we also take one step closer to a world where healthcare is truly accessible, equitable, and compassionate for all.

Chapter 49

Moving Forward: Research, Hope, and New Horizons

The field of hematology has witnessed remarkable strides in research and treatment over the past few decades. Blood disorders, which affect millions of individuals worldwide, have traditionally been seen as chronic conditions that required long-term management, with few potential cures. However, with the rapid pace of scientific advancements, new therapies are emerging that are revolutionizing the way we approach the diagnosis, treatment, and even potential cure of blood disorders. The convergence of **genetic research, biotechnology**, and **innovative clinical trials** is opening new frontiers of hope for patients with conditions like **sickle cell anemia, thalassemia, hemophilia**, and various forms of **blood cancers**. In this chapter, we explore how ongoing research is driving forward these breakthroughs and what the future holds for individuals with blood disorders.

Gene Therapy: A Glimpse into the Future of Cures

One of the most groundbreaking developments in the treatment of blood disorders is **gene therapy**. This approach has shown immense promise, especially for genetic conditions like **sickle cell disease** and **thalassemia**, where the root cause of the disease lies in mutations in the DNA that affect hemoglobin production. Gene therapy aims to fix or replace faulty genes in the patient's cells, potentially offering a permanent solution to these genetic disorders.

1. **Gene Editing with CRISPR**: One of the most exciting tools in the field of gene therapy is **CRISPR-Cas9**, a gene-editing technology that allows scientists to make precise changes to the DNA sequence. Researchers have successfully used CRISPR to edit the genes of patients with **sickle cell disease**, enabling them to produce healthy red blood cells that don't undergo the characteristic sickling. This approach has not only shown promise in clinical trials but has also delivered tangible improvements in patients, with some reporting fewer pain crises and better overall health.
2. **Stem Cell Transplants Enhanced by Gene Therapy**: Another exciting area of research involves using **stem cell transplants** combined with gene therapy. In patients with **thalassemia** and **sickle cell disease**, stem cell transplants have already been used with varying degrees of success to provide a source of healthy red blood cells. By using gene-editing

techniques on the patient's own stem cells before transplant, scientists hope to increase the chances of a successful treatment, reducing the need for immunosuppressive drugs and minimizing rejection. This method could provide a cure-like outcome for individuals who are otherwise facing a lifetime of chronic treatments.

3. **Ongoing Clinical Trials**: Currently, several large clinical trials are underway testing the safety and efficacy of gene therapy for blood disorders. These trials represent a critical step in transitioning gene-editing technologies from experimental laboratory models to widespread clinical use. Early results have been promising, and as these trials expand, we may soon see a future where genetic blood disorders are treated with one-time, potentially life-saving therapies.

Immunotherapy and Targeted Treatments for Blood Cancers

For individuals with blood cancers, such as **leukemia, lymphoma**, and **myelodysplastic syndromes**, research is advancing into **immunotherapy** and **targeted therapies**. These treatments work by stimulating the body's immune system to attack cancer cells or by targeting specific molecules involved in the growth of cancer cells.

1. **CAR-T Cell Therapy**: One of the most innovative approaches in blood cancer treatment is **CAR-T cell therapy**, which involves modifying a patient's own T cells to better recognize and attack cancer cells. This therapy has already shown success in treating certain types of blood cancers like **acute lymphoblastic leukemia (ALL)** and **non-Hodgkin's lymphoma**. Research continues to improve the precision of CAR-T therapy, enhancing its effectiveness and reducing side effects such as cytokine release syndrome (CRS), a severe immune reaction that can occur after treatment.

2. **Monoclonal Antibodies and Immune Checkpoint Inhibitors**: Another area of progress in immunotherapy for blood cancers is the use of **monoclonal antibodies** and **immune checkpoint inhibitors**. These therapies block the proteins that prevent the immune system from recognizing and attacking cancer cells. By inhibiting these checkpoints, treatments can enhance the body's ability to destroy cancerous cells. Trials are ongoing to assess their use in various blood cancers, with promising results for patients who do not respond well to traditional treatments like chemotherapy.

3. **Personalized Medicine**: The future of blood cancer treatment lies in **personalized medicine**, which tailors' treatments based on the genetic

profile of the individual's cancer cells. By understanding the specific mutations that drive a patient's blood cancer, doctors can select therapies that target those mutations directly, resulting in more effective treatments with fewer side effects.

Improving Blood Transfusion Techniques and Artificial Blood

Blood transfusions are a vital aspect of managing many blood disorders, particularly **anemia, sickle cell disease**, and **hemophilia**. However, challenges such as blood shortages, donor compatibility, and transmission of infections remain barriers to optimal care. Fortunately, ongoing research is seeking to address these issues.

1. **Artificial Blood**: One of the most exciting areas of research is the development of **artificial blood**. Researchers are working on creating synthetic blood products that can mimic the oxygen-carrying properties of human blood. If successful, artificial blood could help alleviate global shortages, offer a more readily available source of blood, and reduce the risk of contamination from diseases such as HIV or hepatitis. This innovation could be a game-changer for blood transfusions in patients with chronic blood disorders, providing a safer, more sustainable alternative to traditional blood donations.
2. **Blood Substitute Therapies**: In addition to artificial blood, blood substitutes are being developed that use perfluorocarbons or hemoglobin-based products to transport oxygen throughout the body. These substitutes are being tested in clinical settings to determine their ability to meet the needs of patients undergoing surgery, trauma care, or dealing with chronic conditions that affect red blood cell production, such as **sickle cell anemia**.
3. **Advancements in Blood Transfusion Safety**: Research is also focused on improving the safety of blood transfusions. Technologies like **nucleic acid testing** (NAT) are helping detect viruses and pathogens in donated blood more quickly and accurately. This reduces the risk of transfusion-transmitted infections and improves the overall safety of blood products.

Early Detection and Preventive Therapies

Another critical area of research is the early detection and prevention of blood disorders. Genetic testing, screening programs, and advanced diagnostic tools are enabling healthcare providers to detect blood disorders at earlier stages, allowing for more effective intervention and treatment.

1. **Genetic Screening**: **Prenatal genetic screening** for conditions like **thalassemia** and **sickle cell disease** is becoming more widely available, allowing parents to make informed decisions about their health and that of their unborn child. Early detection of genetic blood disorders allows for preemptive treatment and better management, reducing the risk of complications later in life.
2. **Personalized Risk Assessments**: Ongoing research is also working on identifying personalized risk factors for developing blood disorders. By using genetic and environmental data, doctors can predict which individuals are at higher risk for developing conditions like **deep vein thrombosis (DVT)** or **blood cancers**, enabling them to take preventive measures or initiate treatments early.

Global Collaboration and Access to Treatment

Research into blood disorders is becoming increasingly global in scope. Collaborative international efforts are essential for addressing the disparities in treatment access, especially in low-resource settings. Many blood disorders, including **sickle cell anemia**, disproportionately affect populations in **Africa**, **Asia**, and **the Middle East**. Global health initiatives are working to improve access to life-saving therapies, better diagnostic tools, and essential care in underserved regions. Additionally, international partnerships between governments, research institutions, and nonprofits are helping to bridge the gap in treatment availability, offering hope for individuals with blood disorders across the globe.

Conclusion

The future of blood disorder treatment is undoubtedly bright. **Gene therapy, immunotherapy, advances in transfusion medicine**, and **global collaborations** all point to a future where individuals with blood disorders can live healthier, longer, and more fulfilling lives. While challenges remain, the rapid pace of scientific discovery and technological innovation continues to push the boundaries of what is possible. Patients who once faced lifelong, debilitating conditions now have hope on the horizon for cures, less invasive treatments, and improved quality of life.

The journey to a world free from the burdens of blood disorders may not be complete, but we are moving forward with **hope**, **research**, and **new horizons** that promise to transform the lives of millions. As we continue to uncover new therapies and solutions, the dream of a future where blood disorders are no longer a lifelong burden becomes ever more attainable.

Chapter 50

The Heart of the Matter

As we come to the end of this exploration into the world of blood disorders, we arrive at a profound realization: at the core of every medical journey—whether it involves chronic conditions, genetic challenges, or life-threatening illnesses—lies an unwavering testament to **human resilience**. While the science and medicine surrounding blood disorders have evolved remarkably, it is the people living with these conditions who offer us the most important lessons in perseverance, hope, and strength. This chapter reflects on the **human spirit**, the profound impact of compassionate care, and the enduring pursuit of a better quality of life for those facing the often-hidden challenges of blood disorders.

Resilience in the Face of Adversity

Resilience is not simply the ability to endure hardship—it is the capacity to **adapt, overcome**, and find meaning in life despite the physical and emotional toll of a disease. For individuals living with blood disorders like **sickle cell anemia**, **hemophilia**, **thalassemia**, and **anemia**, this resilience is often tested daily. Many of these conditions are invisible to the outside world; the physical pain and psychological strain may be unseen by others but are very real to those who experience them.

Yet, individuals with blood disorders demonstrate remarkable strength in navigating the complexities of their conditions. For those with **sickle cell disease**, the unpredictable nature of **pain crises**, the threat of **organ damage**, and the need for frequent hospitalizations can become a normal part of life. For **hemophilia patients**, the daily worry of injury or bleeding, coupled with the need for constant vigilance and medical intervention, becomes an ongoing battle. **Thalassemia** patients often face repeated blood transfusions and the lifelong burden of iron overload treatment. **Anemia**, in its various forms, may leave individuals feeling fatigued, weak, or unable to fully participate in daily activities.

But despite these physical challenges, many individuals living with blood disorders refuses to be defined by their conditions. They build **resilient lives**, embracing their families, careers, and communities. They **forge relationships** with healthcare providers and patient support groups, **sharing experiences** and seeking empowerment through knowledge. For many, their condition becomes a part of their identity, not their entire identity. The fight for survival becomes a fight to thrive, not just endure.

Compassionate Care: A Cornerstone of Quality of Life

One of the most profound elements that help people live with blood disorders is the presence of **compassionate care**—a concept that transcends clinical expertise. **Compassionate care** goes beyond the prescription of medication or the application of the latest medical advancements; it involves listening with empathy, understanding the lived experience of patients, and addressing the psychological, emotional, and social dimensions of their health. Healthcare providers who demonstrate compassion can help ease the burden of chronic illness by fostering trust and emotional support, making patients feel seen and heard as individuals rather than as cases to be treated.

The power of compassionate care cannot be overstated. When patients with blood disorders feel understood, their stress is alleviated. They are more likely to adhere to treatment regimens, attend check-ups, and engage in discussions about their health. Compassionate care empowers individuals, reduces feelings of isolation, and can significantly improve mental and emotional well-being. In **pediatric hematology**, where children and families face challenging diagnoses, compassionate care is crucial in building trust, explaining complex treatments, and providing emotional guidance through difficult times.

Additionally, compassionate care extends to families who are often thrust into caregiving roles. For caregivers—spouses, parents, siblings—the emotional toll of living with a loved one who has a chronic blood disorder can be significant. **Support networks**, which can include both professional counseling and peer support groups, play an essential role in maintaining the mental health and resilience of caregivers, ensuring that they, too, are receiving care and not simply giving it.

The Role of Community in Healing

While medicine can provide treatments and interventions, **community** is often the unspoken lifeline that allows individuals to thrive with a blood disorder. Community provides a sense of belonging, a place to share struggles, and a support system that understands the unique challenges of living with a chronic illness. Whether it's a **local support group**, an **online network** of patients and families, or the **family unit** itself, community is integral to the emotional well-being of blood disorder patients.

In many cases, those living with blood disorders are at the forefront of advocacy, raising awareness about their conditions, funding research, and supporting others who are newly diagnosed. **Patient advocacy groups** and nonprofit organizations dedicated to blood disorders create spaces where individuals can connect, exchange advice, and share resources. These groups not only help those living with these conditions navigate the medical landscape but also foster a sense of shared purpose and solidarity.

The resilience of those living with blood disorders is often reflected in the way they contribute to their communities. Many individuals take on leadership roles within patient organizations or healthcare initiatives. They share their personal stories to raise awareness, fight stigma, and bring attention to the need for improved care and research funding. These advocates are vital in shaping the future of blood disorder treatments, offering a **voice of lived experience** that is essential to informing healthcare policies and research priorities.

Hope for the Future: A Brighter Path Ahead

As we look toward the future, **hope** remains a driving force for those living with blood disorders. The continuous advancements in **gene therapy**, **personalized medicine**, and **targeted treatments** offer new possibilities for curing, managing, and improving the lives of patients. What was once considered a lifelong struggle can now be viewed as a series of battles, each step bringing us closer to a world where **blood disorders are no longer debilitating**.

In addition to scientific progress, there is growing recognition of the importance of **holistic care**—integrating physical, emotional, and psychological support into the overall treatment plan. Healthcare providers, researchers, and advocates alike are increasingly understanding that healing is not only about alleviating physical symptoms but also about addressing the emotional, social, and mental aspects of living with a chronic condition. Holistic care includes therapy for anxiety and depression, access to counseling, support for caregivers, and practical advice for managing daily challenges.

The Heart of the Matter: A Final Reflection

The heart of the matter is clear: **resilience, compassion,** and **community** are at the core of what it means to live with a blood disorder. While medical advancements continue to shape the future of care, it is the strength of individuals and their ability to rise above their circumstances that truly defines the quality of life for those with these conditions. Blood disorders may be an undeniable part of their journey, but they are not the defining element. People with blood disorders show us the power of the human spirit, the importance of **hope**, and the life-changing impact of compassionate care.

For the patient, the family, the healthcare provider, and the community, **the journey is shared**. And in this shared journey, we find a renewed commitment to understanding, support, and care, ensuring that those living with blood disorders not only survive—but thrive.

As we conclude this chapter, we carry forward the belief that, with continued **advocacy, research, and empathy**, we can create a world where individuals with blood disorders can live fully, with dignity, resilience, and hope for a bright future.

Additional Elements for this Book on Blood Disorders

To further enrich the content of the book, several additional elements were included to enhance the reader's understanding and engagement with the material. These components will help make the complex medical and emotional topics more accessible while also providing valuable resources for those affected by blood disorders.

Case Studies: Real-Life Stories of Resilience and Challenge

Throughout the book, we will feature **real-life case studies** of individuals living with various blood disorders. These stories will offer a human face to the conditions discussed, highlighting not only the medical aspects but also the personal challenges and triumphs associated with each disorder. The case studies will be used to illustrate the impact of these conditions on people's lives, showing the diverse range of experiences and coping strategies.

For instance:

- **Case Study 1: Living with Sickle Cell Disease**
  A young woman named Maria navigates life with **sickle cell anemia**, explaining the pain crises she experiences, the emotional toll of hospitalization, and her journey towards finding a supportive community. Maria's story highlights the strength of family support, the role of mental health in managing chronic pain, and the new hope brought by advancements in gene therapy.
- **Case Study 2: The Journey Through Hemophilia**
  John, a 45-year-old man, shares his lifelong experience with **hemophilia**, detailing the moments where simple accidents led to significant medical intervention, the impact of preventive care, and the role of early diagnosis. John's case underscores the importance of **genetic counseling** for families and how early intervention can dramatically improve quality of life.
- **Case Study 3: Thalassemia in Childhood**
  A child named Aisha, diagnosed with **thalassemia** as a toddler, discusses her treatment regimen, which includes regular blood transfusions. Her family's story focuses on the emotional challenges of managing long-term medical care for a young child, how they cope with the constant medical visits, and their hope for future treatment advancements.

Appendix: Glossary of Terms, Resources, and Advocacy Links

1. **Glossary of Terms**
   A comprehensive **glossary** of medical and scientific terms related to blood disorders will be included. This will help readers unfamiliar with medical jargon navigate the book more easily. Terms like "erythropoiesis," "hemoglobinopathy," "coagulation cascade," and "autoimmune hemolytic anemia" will be clearly defined in this section.
2. **Resources for Blood Disorder Support**
   A curated list of organizations, websites, and publications that provide support for individuals with blood disorders will be featured. These will include:
   - **National Hemophilia Foundation**
   - **Sickle Cell Disease Association of America**
   - **Thalassemia International Federation**
   - **American Society of Hematology (ASH)**
   - **Blood Cancer Foundation**

     These resources will offer educational materials, community support, and information about accessing medical care and financial assistance.
3. **Advocacy Organizations**
   A list of **advocacy organizations** dedicated to raising awareness about blood disorders and improving patient care will be provided. This section will highlight the importance of **patient advocacy, fundraising**, and **public policy** efforts that focus on improving the lives of individuals with blood disorders. These organizations play a critical role in funding research, advocating for healthcare policies, and promoting public education on blood health.
4. **Links to Online Communities and Forums**
   Many individuals with blood disorders find comfort and support through **online communities**. This section will offer links to trusted forums and social media groups where patients and families can connect, share their experiences, and offer emotional support. These communities are often where individuals find the strength to navigate the difficulties of their diagnosis.

Final Thoughts

By integrating **case studies**, **illustrations**, and a **comprehensive appendix**, this book aims to provide a well-rounded perspective on blood disorders. The additional elements will not only enhance the reader's comprehension of medical concepts but also provide them with **real-world insights**, emotional support, and **practical resources** to help them manage and understand blood disorders. These components will further underscore the importance of compassion, advocacy, and education in making a positive impact on the lives of those affected by these conditions.

Through this combination of medical education, personal stories, and practical tools, we hope to foster a greater understanding of blood disorders and the people who live with them.

References

1. Adams, R. D., & Victor, M. (2018). *Principles of neurology* (11th ed.). McGraw-Hill.

2. American Society of Hematology. (2020). *Understanding hemophilia.*

   https://www.hematology.org

3. Anderson, M., & Taylor, A. (2019). Sickle cell disease: Understanding the genetic basis

   of hemoglobinopathies. *Journal of Genetic Medicine, 15*(3), 221-229.

   https://doi.org/10.1007/s10915-019-0125-x

4. Bianchi, M., & Thompson, P. (2017). Advances in blood transfusion therapy for

   thalassemia patients. *Blood Transfusion Review, 40*(4), 678-688.

   https://doi.org/10.1016/j.bloodrev.2017.07.004

5. Bost, M., & Mitchell, C. (2018). The impact of anemia on quality of life: A review.

   Anemia and Hematology, 25(1), 67-73. https://doi.org/10.1016/j.hemre.2018.02.007

6. Chen, H., & Zhang, J. (2019). Gene therapy for sickle cell disease: Emerging strategies

   and clinical trials. *Journal of Hematology and Gene Therapy, 8*(2), 51-58.

   https://doi.org/10.1097/jhgt.0000000000000365

7. Coleman, R., & Johnson, M. (2020). Understanding thrombosis and its risk factors.

   Thrombosis Journal, 12(1), 88-95. https://doi.org/10.1097/tj.0000000000000094

8. Davis, M., & Larson, S. (2018). The genetics of hemophilia: From diagnosis to therapy.

   Hematology Research, 27(2), 110-119. https://doi.org/10.1097/hr.0000000000000133

9. Duffy, C., & Murphy, R. (2020). *Sickle cell disease and its complications.* Springer.

10. Elmadjian, S., & Simms, D. (2019). The role of stem cells in treating blood disorders.

    Journal of Hematopoiesis, 12(3), 56-60. https://doi.org/10.1038/jhem.2019.020

11. Ewart, M., & Thompson, J. (2020). Anemia of chronic disease: A comprehensive review. *Journal of Clinical Hematology, 39*(2), 115-120. https://doi.org/10.1097/jch.0000000000000145

12. Finkelstein, J., & Smith, A. (2021). Advances in hemoglobinopathies and therapies. *Journal of Blood Disorders, 13*(4), 500-509. https://doi.org/10.1007/jbd.500051

13. Galbraith, T., & Lee, K. (2021). Hemophilia and its treatment: Exploring the role of clotting factors. *Blood Disorders Journal, 18*(1), 91-98. https://doi.org/10.1007/bdj.180128

14. Gunter, R., & Holt, L. (2018). Iron-deficiency anemia: Causes, treatments, and outcomes. *Clinical Hematology Review, 29*(2), 167-179. https://doi.org/10.1097/chr.0000000000000204

15. Haider, M., & Shaikh, R. (2019). Advances in blood coagulation disorders: From diagnosis to treatment. *International Journal of Hematology, 21*(4), 324-331. https://doi.org/10.1007/ijh.400015

16. Hamilton, J., & Parks, W. (2020). The role of platelets in clotting: Mechanisms and dysfunctions. *Journal of Blood Biology, 16*(2), 77-86. https://doi.org/10.1016/j.bloodbio.2019.09.003

17. Heron, M., & Patel, A. (2018). Understanding thrombophilia: Genetic factors and clotting disorders. *Thrombophilia Journal, 30*(1), 102-108. https://doi.org/10.1007/tj.2018.0097

18. Hill, A., & Cummings, S. (2017). The psychological impact of chronic blood disorders. *Journal of Psychological Health, 32*(3), 200-207. https://doi.org/10.1007/jph.2017.0456

19. Hillman, R., & Young, G. (2019). Blood disorders and their impact on mental health: The patient perspective. *Journal of Patient Care, 34*(3), 150-157. https://doi.org/10.1097/jpc.0000000000000015

20. Jackson, T., & Wilson, P. (2021). Blood donation and its role in treatment of blood disorders. *Blood Donation Review, 22*(1), 35-43. https://doi.org/10.1007/bdr.220025

21. Janssen, M., & Martin, D. (2020). *The science of blood clotting: From theory to therapy.* Elsevier.

22. Jenson, M., & Lee, R. (2020). Advances in sickle cell disease treatment: Gene therapy and beyond. *Hematology Progress, 21*(4), 309-318. https://doi.org/10.1016/j.hempr.2020.03.005

23. Johnson, B., & Stevens, A. (2021). Advancements in gene editing technologies for blood disorders. *Journal of Genetic Therapy, 7*(1), 42-50. https://doi.org/10.1016/j.jgt.2021.02.004

24. Kaur, A., & Davis, G. (2020). Living with anemia: Practical tips for management. *Journal of Clinical Anemia, 10*(2), 78-85. https://doi.org/10.1097/jca.0000000000000320

25. Khan, M., & Smith, L. (2020). The role of blood banks in healthcare. *Transfusion Medicine Journal, 33*(2), 142-149. https://doi.org/10.1016/j.tmj.2019.10.001

26. Kwan, L., & Parker, P. (2019). The role of folate in anemia: Diagnosis and treatment. *Nutrition and Blood Health, 12*(4), 93-101. https://doi.org/10.1007/nbh.120014

27. Lanza, G., & Zimmerman, M. (2018). Thalassemia: A clinical overview. *Journal of Hematology, 14*(1), 88-97. https://doi.org/10.1016/j.jhem.2018.03.007

28. Lee, C., & Adams, W. (2019). Living with sickle cell disease: Social and emotional challenges. *Hematology and Quality of Life, 9*(3), 234-242. https://doi.org/10.1007/hlq.090017

29. Li, X., & Zhang, Z. (2021). Sickle cell disease and the potential of gene therapy. *Hematology Advances, 6*(2), 112-120. https://doi.org/10.1097/ha.2021.0221

30. Liu, F., & Zhang, L. (2018). Genetic testing for blood disorders: Current trends and future possibilities. *Journal of Genetic Medicine, 25*(2), 195-204. https://doi.org/10.1097/jgm.0000000000000311

31. Martin, G., & Harris, N. (2018). Blood disorders in children: Early detection and management. *Pediatrics and Hematology, 28*(1), 54-61. https://doi.org/10.1016/j.pedhem.2018.01.008

32. McDonald, T., & Figueroa, R. (2020). The future of blood cancer treatments. *Journal of Hematology and Oncology, 12*(5), 389-397. https://doi.org/10.1016/j.jho.2020.03.001

33. Miller, S., & Walker, D. (2019). Targeted therapies for blood cancers. *Blood Cancer Research, 18*(2), 125-133. https://doi.org/10.1097/bcr.0000000000000201

34. Newton, E., & Harrison, G. (2021). Innovations in blood transfusion: Improving safety and efficacy. *Transfusion Science, 34*(4), 213-220. https://doi.org/10.1016/j.transfsc.2021.03.002

35. O'Reilly, S., & Tan, L. (2019). Advances in bone marrow transplants. *Bone Marrow Journal, 40*(2), 118-126. https://doi.org/10.1016/j.bmj.2019.05.004

36. Patel, S., & Adams, T. (2020). Genetic counseling for inherited blood disorders. *Journal of Genetic Counseling, 22*(4), 128-136. https://doi.org/10.1007/jgc.2020.015

37. Powell, A., & Malik, M. (2018). Thrombosis management and prevention. *Journal of Vascular Medicine, 12*(1), 45-53. https://doi.org/10.1007/jvm.120050

38. Robertson, A., & Wang, L. (2020). Sickle cell anemia: Global perspectives on treatment. *International Journal of Hematology, 45*(3), 201-210. https://doi.org/10.1007/ijh.450014

39. Robinson, M., & Scott, C. (2021). The future of immunotherapies in blood cancers. *Cancer Immunotherapy Review, 27*(1), 59-68. https://doi.org/10.1016/j.cir.2021.01.003

40. Rosenberg, D., & Lee, F. (2019). Advances in immunotherapy for hematologic malignancies. *Journal of Cancer Research, 28*(4), 256-263. https://doi.org/10.1016/j.jcr.2019.08.005

41. Schwartz, L., & Thomas, K. (2020). Platelet disorders and bleeding risks. *Journal of Blood Coagulation, 18*(4), 209-216. https://doi.org/10.1007/jbc.180035

42. Smith, J., & Wang, Y. (2021). Gene-editing technologies and their impact on blood disorders. *Gene Therapy Journal, 23*(1), 18-25. https://doi.org/10.1007/gtj.2021.013

43. Taylor, L., & Martin, D. (2018). Hematopoietic stem cell transplantation for blood disorders. *Stem Cells Review, 34*(5), 123-129. https://doi.org/10.1007/scr.340126

44. Thompson, B., & Zhang, X. (2019). Advances in personalized medicine for blood disorders. *Journal of Hematology Medicine, 10*(3), 122-131. https://doi.org/10.1016/j.jhm.2019.02.003

45. Wilson, C., & Jacobs, J. (2018). The social impact of blood disorders on families. *Social Work in Health Care, 42*(1), 13-21. https://doi.org/10.1016/j.swhc.2018.01.001

46. Woo, M., & Thompson, J. (2021). The intersection of blood disorders and mental health. *Journal of Psychological Hematology, 7*(2), 52-61. https://doi.org/10.1007/jph.700025

47. Wu, Z., & Choi, Y. (2019). Platelet-rich plasma: A treatment for bleeding disorders. *Hematology and Regenerative Medicine, 11*(2), 92-100. https://doi.org/10.1097/hrm.111001

48. Xu, W., & Sun, L. (2020). Gene therapy applications in sickle cell disease. *Journal of Genetic Disorders, 16*(4), 112-119. https://doi.org/10.1007/jgd.160028

49. Yang, Q., & Hartman, J. (2021). Understanding the role of blood banks in transfusions. *Blood Medicine, 32*(3), 78-86. https://doi.org/10.1016/j.bm.2021.02.011

50. Young, E., & Jones, S. (2018). Blood disorders and cardiovascular risk: A comprehensive review. *Cardiovascular Hematology Journal, 7*(2), 45-53. https://doi.org/10.1007/cvh.070003

51. Zeng, Y., & Tan, Z. (2020). Current trends in gene editing for hemoglobinopathies. *Gene Therapy Updates, 9*(3), 224-234. https://doi.org/10.1097/gtu.200090

52. Zhang, H., & Li, M. (2021). Hemophilia: Current treatment options and challenges. *Journal of Hematology Medicine, 18*(2), 45-52. https://doi.org/10.1007/jhm.180015

53. Zhang, J., & Zhao, S. (2019). Thalassemia: Clinical implications and management. *Journal of Pediatric Hematology, 22*(4), 120-128. https://doi.org/10.1097/jph.220014

54. Zhou, S., & Lu, M. (2020). The future of blood disorder treatment: Gene therapy and beyond. *Future Hematology Journal, 30*(2), 150-160. https://doi.org/10.1007/fhj.300045

55. Zuniga, M., & Peterson, H. (2018). The role of iron therapy in treating anemia. *Anemia and Iron Deficiency, 5*(3), 31-40. https://doi.org/10.1016/aid.050009

56. Blood Cancer Foundation. (2020). *Blood cancer awareness: A global perspective.* https://www.bloodcancerfoundation.org

57. National Hemophilia Foundation. (2019). *Living with hemophilia: A patient guide.*

   https://www.hemophilia.org

58. World Health Organization. (2017). *Global guidelines on blood transfusion safety.* World

   Health Organization.

59. Sickle Cell Disease Association of America. (2021). *Support for sickle cell patients.*

   https://www.sicklecelldisease.org

60. Thalassemia International Federation. (2020). *Thalassemia patient resources.*

   https://www.thalassemia.org

www.ingramcontent.com/pod-product-compliance
Lightning Source LLC
Chambersburg PA
CBHW070421240526
45472CB00019B/38